Introductory Nutrition

Manual of Basic Nutrition Exercises

Introductory Nutrition
Manual of Basic Nutrition Exercises

Sooja K. Kim, Ph.D., R.D.
Patrice Fraker, M.Ed., R.D.
Department of Home Economics
Bowling Green State University
Bowling Green, Ohio

Bowling Green State University Popular Press
Bowling Green, Ohio 43403

Acknowledgements:

The authors thank the following for permission to reprint:

Krehl and Winters: "Effects of cooking methods on retention of vitamins and minerals in vegetables." Copyright © The American Dietetic Association. Reprinted by permission from *Journal of the American Dietetic Association*, Vol. 26:966, 1950.

From Young, E.A. Update: Nutritional Analysis of Fast Foods, *Dietetic Currents*, 1981. (Ross Laboratories, Columbus, Ohio).

Metropolitan Life Insurance Companies for table entitled "Metropolitan Life Insurance Weight Standards".

Page 3, Table 1.1, *Nutritional Evaluation of Food Processing*, Second Edition, 1977. The AVI Publishing Co., Inc., Westport, CT. 06881.

Library of Congress Catalogue Card No.: 87-71637
ISBN: 0-87972-401-3 pb.

TABLE OF CONTENTS

PREFACE

This manual provided practical applications for nutrition information. Each two-hour lab covers a different aspect of nutrition. The labs provides students with a working knowledge of the calories and nutrients found in foods. Nutrition labeling, anthropometric measurements, and computers provide for new areas in the field of nutrition. Finally, experience in selection and use of food composition handbooks is included.

Suggestions made by users of the original manual "Applied Nutrition Exercises" by Mrs. Betty Mackey have been helpful during the preparation of this manual and are gratefully acknowledged. Students in basic Nutrition and other Foods classes have provided inspiration through their questions, their comments, their needs, and their interests. Their contributions are immeasurable.

We thank the many people who have helped in the preparation of the manuscript: faculty members and graduate teaching assistants in Foods and Nutrition for their generous assistance and understanding; staff at Word Processing Center, Bowling Green State University, who typed this manuscript but, most of all, we acknowledge the inspiration provided by Mrs. Betty Mackey, author of "Applied Nutrition Exercises."

Finally, we wish to thank Mrs. Martha Eckman, former Director of the Technical Writing Program, Bowling Green State University, for her patience, suggestions, and help in completing this endeavor.

APPENDICES

LIST OF ILLUSTRATIONS

LIST OF TABLES AND FORMS

NUTRITION LABORATORY MANUAL

Summary Statement. The following manual provides students with practical experience in applying data to problems in nutrition. Procedures and related data are provided for nine laboratory experiences. Students are expected to have prerequisite knowledge (general chemistry series) before enrolling in Home Economics 307, Nutrition, for which this manual has been prepared.

Introduction and purpose.

The purpose of this laboratory manual is to:

- Provide students with practice in basic nutritional assessment.
- Provide students with a working knowledge of caloric and nutrient values of foods.
- Provide students with practice in location and use of reliabel resource materials for nutrient content.
- Provide students with practice in writing menus that meet the nutritional needs of adults.
- Provide students with a working knowledge of the USRADs for healthy adults.
- Provide students with information and practical applications for nutritional labeling.

In the following pages, you will find a listing of current LABORATORY PRACTICES for general Home Economics Laboratoris. This list of practices will be followed by instructions in use of the balance scale -- a piece of equipment used in all studies of nutrition.

FOOD LABORATORY PRACTICES AND STANDARDS

Personal Appearance

A uniform or full length lab coat must be worn during laboratory period.

This uniform or lab coat should not be worn to other classes.

If only one uniform is to be used, make sure laundry facilities are adequate. Mark your uniform with your name.

Uniforms are to be entirely white. They are to be worn as a dress. No sweaters can be worn over uniforms.

Suitable lingerie must be worn with the uniform.

- Sleeves may be three quarter lenth, or short, but not sleeveless. One or more pockets are desirable.

- Soiled uniforms are not to be worn.

Hair is to be covered with an inconspicuous type of hair net. Provide two nets so if one is lost another is available. Net is to be worn so that most of hair is covered. Put on net before entering laboratory.

- Low heeled shoes are to be worn. Boots and other cold weather or rain footwear are out of place in the laboratory.

- Costume jewelry should not be worn. Take care of rings or watches to avoid losing them.

Personal Property

- Books, pocketbooks, and similar items are to kept in a drawer or cupboard provided in each kitchen for that purpose.

Outer clothing and wraps are to be placed in a closet in the dressing room.

Personal Hygiene

- See that your hands and fingernails are clean before beginning work.

- If it is necessary to touch your face, hair, or handkerchief while cooking, always wash your hands at once.

- Use paper towels for drying your hands.

- Do not sneeze or cough upon food. Avoid placing you handkerchief upon laboratory counters or tables.

Procedures

Method of work in each kitchen:

- Place small equipment on small tray after use. (Soiled spoons, spatulas, etc.)
- Measure all material level and accurately. Hold spatula vertically when leveling material in measuring cup or spoon.
- Handle utensils quietly; keep drawers and cabinet doors closed.
- Keep counters clean and orderly at all times. Soak dishes or pans when first emptied; wipe up any material spilled.
- Use boards or the stainless steel strip for resting hot utensils so as not to mar counter tops.
- Avoid waste; return amy material not used to supply cart; turn off range units when not in use; adjust heat so as to avoid rapid boiling.
- Work from right ot left, with soiled dishes stacked at right of sink, and clean dishes placed temporarily to left of drainer. Store all equipment in correct locations in cabinets.
- Wash dishes in this order: glasses, silver, tableware, cooking utensils.
- Drain dishwater through strainer of sink; remove food particles from drainage cup.

Supply table and carts: (responsibility of class)

- Use small tray for carrying supplies to and from supply cast. Have enough cups, etc., to pick up all supplies at one time.
- Avoid carrying general containers of supplies to your desk. Each student is to wipe up any material spilled.
- Replace covers on supply containers after using (press-down lides must be set on loosely until clean-up time). Be sure to keep covers on baking powder, coffee, and flavorings.
- Return extra dishes, utensils, broken glass, and clean empty cans to the supply cart.
- Use damp dish cloth to wipe off all containers. Make sure whole cart if neat and tidy before whelling cart to pantry.
- Wipe off table tops in display area, and dispose of paper.
- Check individual kitchen drawers, cupboards, range, counter, and sink.
- Check dish towels and dish cloths. Return them to the cart.
- Rub cleanser on stained towels and dish cloths before placing them on the cart.

Care of Equipment

- Thermometers: Remove thermometer from cooking medium or from meat and place the thermometer at back of workspace. Wash and rinse it in water about the same temperature. Dry it. If mercury column has separated, remove the thermometer from kitchen unit and hand to instructor.

- Bread Boards: Cover with pastry cloth and use only for kneading, rolling and cutting out dough. (Large Board)

- Cutting Boards: (Small Boards) Use for chopping vegetables and pouding and cutting meats. Wash the board and rinse it. Dry it. Scrub it with scrub brush if necessary.

- Pastry Cloth: Shake excess flour into a disposer sink, or into paper. Do not shake pastry cloths into wastebasket. If cloth is dry, fold it with flour side in and place on supply cart. If cloth is soiled, place it on a second pile on cart.

- Disposers: Instructor will advise you on starting and stopping disposers. Run cold water in the disposer after the grinding cycle. All food scraps should be disposed of in this manner except bones, seeds, grease, or coffee grounds. Containers will be provided for these scraps.

- Burned Utensils: If food burns in utensil, soak the utensil in detergent and hot water. Use steel wool or SOS pads if necessary.

- Iron Skillets: After washing and drying an iron skillet and lid, store them with lid at a slight angle to prevent rusting. Dry with paper towel and place on warm burner or in over to finish drying.

- Desks: Observe location of dishes and utensils in drawers and cabinets as indicated on cards in each kitchen. Learn proper locations and leave the kitchen as it should be at end of each laboratory (even if you find it otherwise when you come in).

- Silverware: Each kitchen has silverware for meal service. Keep you silverware in a matched set.

- Floor: It anything is spilled, clean it at once; use a paper towel. At end of period, check to see that floor is in good condition. Sweep your kitchen, if necessary.

Dishwashing and Clean-Up

- Preparation for dishwashing: scrape dishes; empty any dishes which are soaking, stack soiled dishes at right of sink.

- Wash all dishes with hot, sudsy water in right compartment; rinse in very hot water in left compartment. Use sanitizing solution in rinse water.

<u>Ranges</u>: (group responsibility)

- Clean all range surfaces (including driptray under burners) with old rags or damp paper towel, dry the surfaces at once with cloth or paper towel. Use scrubbing pads for resistent spots.

- If ovens or broilers are used, see that they are cleaned when cooled.

- Check to see that all burners and switches are turned off.

- Each kitchen group is responsible for the appearance of its range(s).

Do not leave laboratory until dismissed by instructor.
All students are responsible for condition of laboratory at the end of the period.
Each kitchen will be graded occasionally.

USING THE BALANCE SCALE

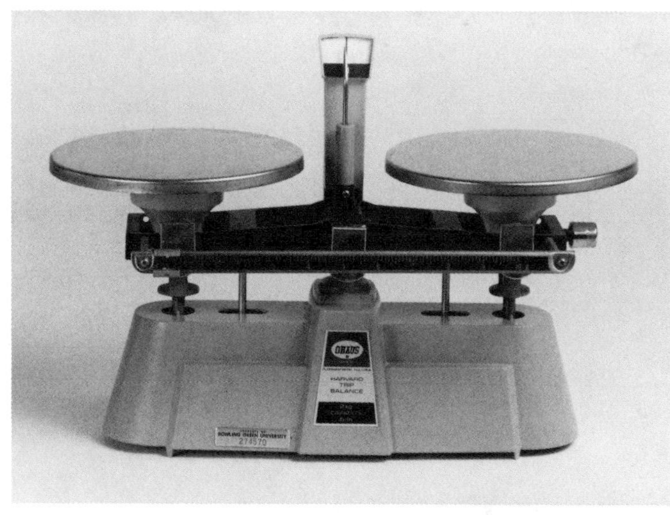

A. Safety Stopper

B. Balance Pans

C. Zero Adjustment Knob

D. Zero Balance Indicator

E. Slide Weight

Figure 1. The Harvard Trip Balance

1. The balance scale is a delicate instrument. It should be carried with two hands. The rubber safety stoppers should be in place whenever the scale is moved.

2. To use the scale, remove the rubber stoppers.

3. Return the slide weight to zero.

4. Check to see if the empty scale is balanced at the zero point. If the indicator is not on zero when the scale is empty, adjust the zero adjustment knob under the right balance pan.

5. Protect the surface of the balance pans with plastic wrap.

6. Place the food item to be measured on the left balance pan. Add weights to the right side of the scale until the balance pan is close to zero.

7. Make the final weight adjustment by moving the slide weight to the right until the indicator is on zero.

8. Total the grams of weight on the right balance pan and add this to the weight indicated by the slide weight to get a final reading.

9. Remove the weights and the food at the same time to prevent the scale from being damaged.

LESSON 1

Food and Its Relation to Health: Dietary Assessment and Anthropometric Measures

Objectives:

Upon completion of the lesson, the student will be able to:

- Complete a dietary self evaluation
- Select and correctly use the appropriate food composition reference books
- Identify important food sources for the major nutrients
- Make recommendations for dietary improvement based on calculation of dietary intake records
- Identify important food sources for the major nutrients
- Describe and discuss specified anthropometric measures as a tool of nutrition assessment.

Equipment and Materials:

Bathroom Scale
Calipers (Lange, USA)
Tape Measure
USDA: Food Composition Handbooks: Nos. 8-1 through 8-9, 72, 456.
Pennington, and Church, H. *Food Value of Portions Commonly Used*, Philadelphia: J.B. Lippincott, 1980.
Frisancho, A.R. "Triceps Skin Fold and Upper Arm Muscle Size Norms for Assessment of Nutritional Status," 27: 1052-58, 1974. (Refer to the Textbook by Robinson and Lamler, *Normal and Therapeutic Nutrition*, New York, 16th ed., MacMillan, 1982, pp. 794, 795.)

Procedure:

Twice during this course a diet assessment and anthropometric measurements will be taken.

A. A dietary assessment will consist of:
   1. 2 Day Diet Intake Record
   2. Calculation of Nutrient Content
   3. Changes Needed to Correct or Improve Deficiencies

B. Anthropometrics are physical measurements. The following measures will be taken:
   1. Height
   2. Weight
   3 Elbow Measurement (used to estimate frame size)
   4. Mid-Arm Circumference (used to estimate muscle stores)
   5. Triceps Skinfold Measurement (used to estimate fat stores and to calculate estimated muscle stores)

How to Complete a Dietary Intake Record

1. Record everything you eat and drink (excluding water) for a two day time period. Include one weekend day in the record.

2. Describe your food intake as accurately as possible. For example: 2% milk, whole wheat bread, casserole with noodles, tuna, milk.

3. Record the amounts eaten in common measurements. Be Exact. For example: 8 oz. cup of orange juice made from frozen concentrate, 1/2 of a 3 inch diameter Delicious apple. Food portions are often underestimated. It is important to record the amounts accurately. If necessary, take a set of measuring spoons and cups with you!

4. If you are taking any food or vitamin or mineral supplement, record the content of the supplement and the frequency of use on a separate sheet of paper.

How to Take Anthropometric Measurements

1. Take the height measurement by having the person stand with his/her back straight and feet against the wall. Take height in stocking feet. Record in inches and centimeters.

2. Take the actual weight by using a bathroom scale (a pedestel scale is usually more accurate if one is available). Record the weight in pounds and kilograms.

3. Using the Metropolitan Life Insurance Weight Standards reference in the appendix, determine your frame size. Record the elbow measurement and your frame size.

4. The arm circumference is measured at the midpoint of the arm between the elbow and the olecranon process. The olecranon process is the prominent bone at the end of each shoulder. Use a tape meaure to determine the midpoint and mark with the tip of a marker (bare arms or short sleeves work out best!) The arm circumference measurement should then be made at the midpoint with the arm relaxed and hanging by one's side. The tape should measure firmly around the arm but should not cause an indentation. If the measurement is made in inches, convert to centimeters by multiplying by 2.5 and record (in centimeters).

5. The triceps skinfold measurement is taken at the midpoint of the arm which should be relaxed and hanging by one's side. The person taking the measurement should stand behind the subject and pinch a layer of skin and fat vertically away from the arm muscle. The calipers should be positioned in an open stance above the skinfold. The lever should then be released on the calipers so that they grasp the skinfold and fat. Read the value on the caliper dial. Take two more readings, average the values, and record <u>only</u> the average value on Table 5. If using plastic calipers, see your instructor for directions.

6. Arm muscle circumference is a calculated value and will be done in the evaluation section.

Evaluation:

Anthropometric Measures

1. Use the actual height and weight values obtained to compare with several ideal weight values and the American average.

   A. Metropolitan Life Insurance Weight Standards: These "ideal" weight standards are based on frame size and lowest mortality for Americans. Use the reference in appendix to determine your "ideal" weight according to this method. Record and compare your weight against this standard on Table 5.

   B. Height squared method: This is an "ideal" weight formula that correlates body mass with the degree of fatness. First, convert height in centimeters to meters by dividing by 100. Example: 180 cm ÷ 100 = 1.8. Second, square the height in meters. Example: 1.8 x 1.8 = 3.2. Third, use the following formulas:

      Men: Ht. in meters^2 x 22.4 = Ideal Weight in Kilograms
      Women: Ht. in meters^2 x 20.9 = Ideal Weight in Kilograms

      Calculate your ideal weight according to this formula and record. Then compare your ideal with your actual weight on Table 5.

   C. Simple Formula: This "ideal" formula is used for rapid evaluations in mnay health care institutions. Use the following formulas:

      Men: 110 lb. for the 1st 5 feet of height
      Add 5 pounds for each additional inch of height
      Women: 100 lb. for the 1st 5 feet of height
      Add 5 pounds for each addtiional inch of height

   D. USA "Average" Weights: These weigths are based on data obtained by the DHEW in the Hanes Study, 1971-1974. Refer to the data in the appendix to determine what the DHEW found to be the average American weight for your height and sex. Compare your weight and complete Table 5.

2. Determine the norm for Mid Arm: Circumference (MAC) and triceps (TSF) skinfolds for your sex by referring to the data on pp. 794-795 in the textbook Normal and Therapeutic Nutrition. Record the norms and compare with your actual values by completing the appropriate sections of Table 5.

3. Use the textbook by Robinson and Lawler, Normal and Therapeutic Nutrition, and record the norm for mid arm muscle circumference (MAMC) values. Use the following formula to determine your estimated mid arm muscle circumference:

   MAMC(cm) = MAC(cm) - [3.14 x TSF(cm)]

   Determine your mid arm muscle circumference and compare to the norm on Table 5.

Dietary Intake

1. Use a separate food intake sheet for each day. Group like foods together (if consumed on the same day) and list them on the sheets.

2. Consult the food composition books to calculate the nutritive value for the quantity of food you ate. Record the nutrient values in the appropriate spaces.

3. Total each column to get your intake for one day.

4. Complete the Summary of Nutrient Intake chart.

   a. Record the daily totals of each nutrient in the approriate spaces. Average the two day intake for each nutrient and record this.
   b. Record the RDA's for your age and sex. Note whether your nutrient intake was above or below the RDA and what the difference was. Record this information.
      Example: ± Difference ± 20 mg.
   c. Indicate which nutrients are below the RDA by making a checkmark (√) in the appropriate space. Indicate which nutrients are below two-thirds (0-66% of RDA) of the RDA by making a checkmark (√) in the appropriate space.

5. Complete the Summary of Protein, Energy, Carbohydrate, and Fat Intake. Calculate the percent of your diet derived from protein, fat, and carbohydrate. Determine the % of protein derived from animal sources.

6. Evaluate your food intake by completing the Food Selection Score Card. Record your daily score and your average score.

   Select one of the days of your food intake record and decide what food items you could add or change to get a 100% score on the Food Selection Card. Note, in writing, on the bottom of the Food Selection Score Card exactly what foods you would change or add to accomplish this.

7. Complete the bar graph which indicates how your diet compares to the RDA standards.

Table 1.

Analysis of Dietary Intake (Initial week)

Date (Day 1)

Food	Measure of Serving	Wt. Gm.	Cal-ories Kcal.	Pro-tein Gm.	Fat Gm.	Carbo-hy-drate Gm.	Ca mg.	Na mg.	Fe mg.	Vitamin A I.U.	Thia-mine mg.	Ribo-flavin mg.	Nia-cin mg.	Ascorbic Acid mg.
Total														
RDA (1980)														
%RDA														

Table 1. (continued)

Analysis of Dietary Intake (Initial week)

Date (Day 2)

Food	Measure of Serving	Wt. Gm.	Cal-ories Kcal.	Pro-tein Gm.	Fat Gm.	Carbo-hy-drate Gm.	Ca mg.	Na mg.	Fe mg.	Vitamin A I.U.	Thia-mine mg.	Ribo-flavin mg.	Nia-cin mg.	Ascorbic Acid mg.
Total														
RDA (1980)								X						
%RDA								X						

Table 2.

Analysis of Dietary Intake (Final week)

Date (Day 1)

Food	Measure of Serving	Wt. Gm.	Cal-ories Kcal.	Pro-tein Gm.	Fat Gm.	Carbo-hy-drate Gm.	Ca mg.	Na mg.	Fe mg.	Vitamin A I.U.	Thia-mine mg.	Ribo-flavin mg.	Nia-cin mg.	Ascorbic Acid mg.
Total														
RDA (1980)														
%RDA														

Table 2. (continued)

Analysis of Dietary Intake (Final week)

Date (Day 2)

Food	Measure of Serving	Wt. Gm.	Cal- ories Kcal.	Pro- tein Gm.	Fat Gm.	Carbo- hy- drate Gm.	Ca mg.	Na mg.	Fe mg.	Vitamin A I.U.	Thia- mine mg.	Ribo- flavin mg.	Nia- cin mg.	Ascorbic Acid mg.
Total														
RDA (1980)								X						
%RDA								X						

Table 3.
SUMMARY OF NUTRIENT INTAKE
MINERALS AND VITAMINS

(Initial Week)

	Calcium mg	Thiamin mg	Riboflavin mg	Iron mg	Niacin mg	Vit. A mg	Vit. C mg	Sodium mg
Day 1								
Day 2								
Average								
RDA								
±Difference								
Less than RDA								
LESS than 2/3 RDA								

Table 4.
SUMMARY OF NUTRIENT INTAKE
ENERGY, PROTEIN, CARBOHYDRATE AND FAT

(Initial Week)

	Energy kcal	Protein			Carbohydrate				
		Total gm	Animal gm	Plant gm	Total gm	Starch gm	Sugar[a] gm	Sugar[b] gm	Fat gm
Day 1									
Day 2									
Average									
RDA		c							d
% of kcal[e]									

a. From milk and fruit.

b. From added sugar.

c. RDA for protein equals your weight in kg x 0.8 gm.

d. Multiply gm of protein, carbohydrate and fat by the factors 4, 4 and 9, respectively.

e. Divide by the dietary calories and then multiply by 100.

Table 3.
SUMMARY OF NUTRIENT INTAKE
MINERALS AND VITAMINS

(Final Week)

	Calcium mg	Thiamin mg	Riboflavin mg	Iron mg	Niacin mg	Vit. A mg	Vit. C mg	Sodium mg
Day 1								
Day 2								
Average								
RDA								
±Difference								
Less than RDA								
Less than 2/3 RDA								

Table 4.
SUMMARY OF NUTRIENT INTAKE
ENERGY, PROTEIN, CARBOHYDRATE AND FAT

(Final Week)

	Energy kcal	Protein			Carbohydrate				Fat gm
		Total gm	Animal gm	Plant gm	Total gm	Starch gm	Sugar[a] gm	Sugar[b] gm	
Day 1									
Day 2									
Average									
RDA	c	d			d				d
% of kcal[e]									

a. From milk and fruit.

b. From added sugar.

c. RDA for protein equals your weight in kg x 0.8 gm.

d. Multiply gm of protein, carbohydrate and fat by the factors 4, 4 and 9, respectively.

e. Divide by the dietary calories and then multiply by 100.

Anthropometrics

Height ________ inches = ________ cm

Elbow Measure _______ inches   Frame size ________

"Ideal" Weight by Metropolitan Life Chart _______   Mid Arm Circumference Norm ________

"Ideal" Weight by Height Squared Method _______   Triceps Skinfold Norm ________

"Ideal" Weight by a Simple Method _______   Mid Arm Muscle Circum. Norm________

"Average" Weight of Americans for Height/Age/Sex ________

Table 5
Arthropometrics Comparison

Anthropometric Measures:	Initial Week Date	Mid-Course* Date	Final Week Date
ACTUAL WEIGHT			
% of Ideal[1]			
% of Ideal[2]			
% of Ideal[3]			
% of Average[4]			
ACTUAL MID ARM CIRCUMFERENCE			
% of Norm			
ACTUAL TRICEPS SKINFOLD MEASURE			
% of Norm			
MID ARM MUSCLE CALCULATION			
% of Norm			

* Optional by Student

[1] Metropolitan Life Chart Value

[2] Height Squared Formula Value

[3] Simple Formula Value

[4] Average American Value for Height/Age/Sex

Table 6.

FOOD SELECTION SCORE CARD

Food Group	Amounts Recommended	Food	Points	Your Daily Score: Initial Wk. Day 1	Initial Wk. Day 2	Final Wk. Day 1	Final Wk. Day 2
Milk[1]	2 cups or more	2 cups	25				
		1 cup					
Meat[2]	2 servings or more	2 servings, including at least 1 of meat, poultry, or fish	25				
		1 serving of any of above	15				
		1 serving of another food in meat group	10				
Vegetable-Fruit[3]	4 servings or more	1 serving of citrus fruit	10				
		1 serving of dark-green or deep-yellow vegetable	10				
		2 servings of any fruit or vegetable	10				
Bread-Cereal[4]	4 servings more	4 servings	20				
		3 servings	15				
		2 servings	10				
		1 serving	5				
TOTAL SCORE							
			Average[5]				

[1]Milk group: maximal score 25
1 cup = 8 oz. of milk
Equivalents in calcium value:
1" cube of cheddar-type cheese--2/3 cup of milk
1/2 cup of cottage cheese--1/3 cup of milk
2 tablespoons of cream cheese--1 tablespoon of milk
1/2 cup of ice cream--1/4 cup of milk

[2]Meat Group: maximal score 25
1 serving - 2 to 3 oz. of lean, cooked meet, poultry, or fish, all without bone
1 serving - 2 eggs
2 servings - 1 cup of cooked, dry beans, dry peas, or lentils
1 serving - 4 tablespoons of peanut butter

[3]Vegetable-Fruit Group: maximal score 30
1 serving - 1/2 cup of vegetable or fruit of an ordinary size serving

[4]Bread-Cereal Group: maximal score 20
1 serving - 1 slice of bread
1 serving - 1 ounce ready-to-eat cereal
1 serving - 1/2 to 3/4 cup of cooked cereal, rice, macaroni, or cornmeal

[5]Calculate the average by adding the two "Total Scores" and dividing by two.

Note: No more than the maximal score for each group may be credited daily.

Form 1.

Charting Your Nutrient Intake
(Initial Week)

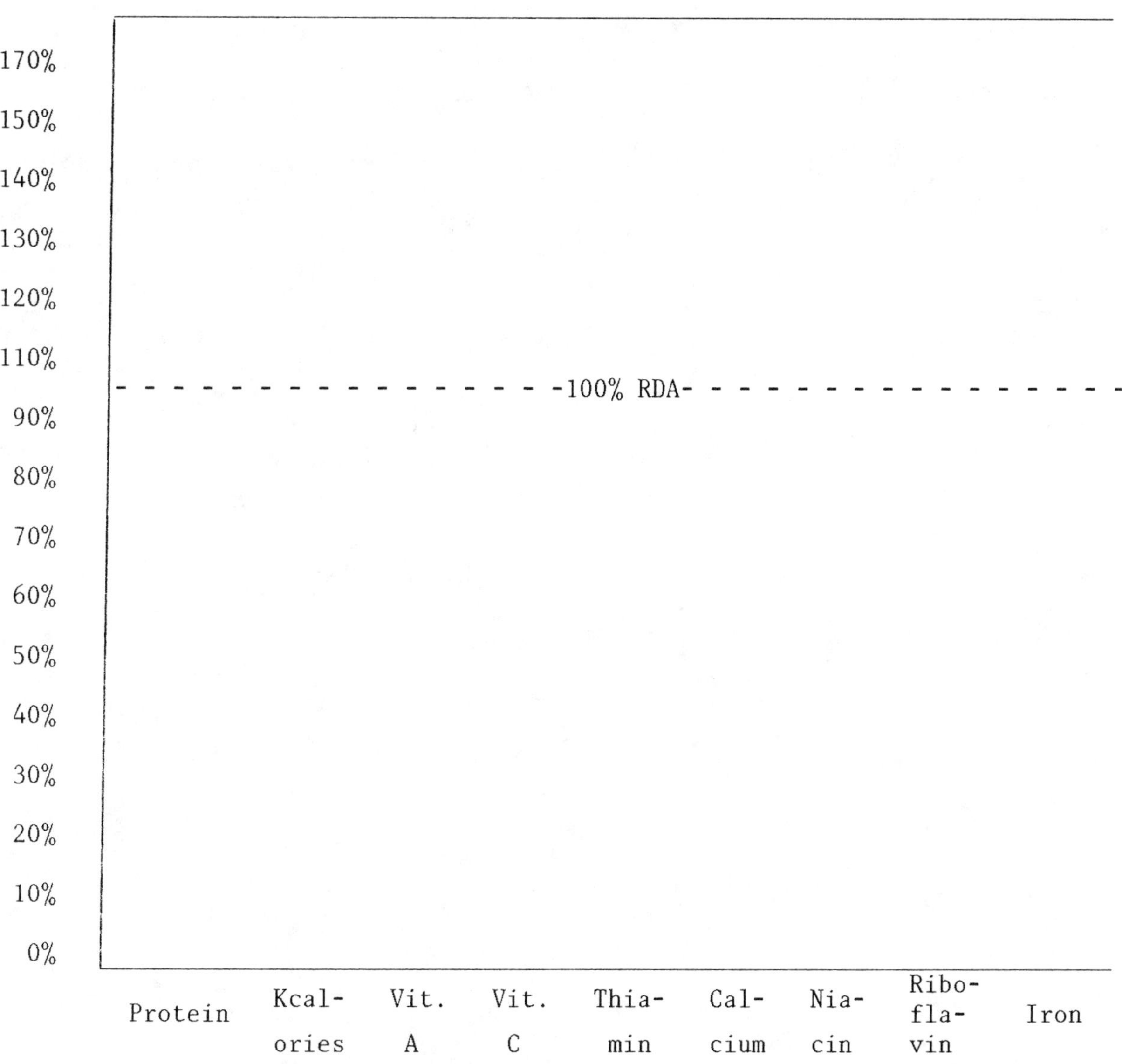

Form 1. (continued)

Charting Your Nutrient Intake
(Final Week)

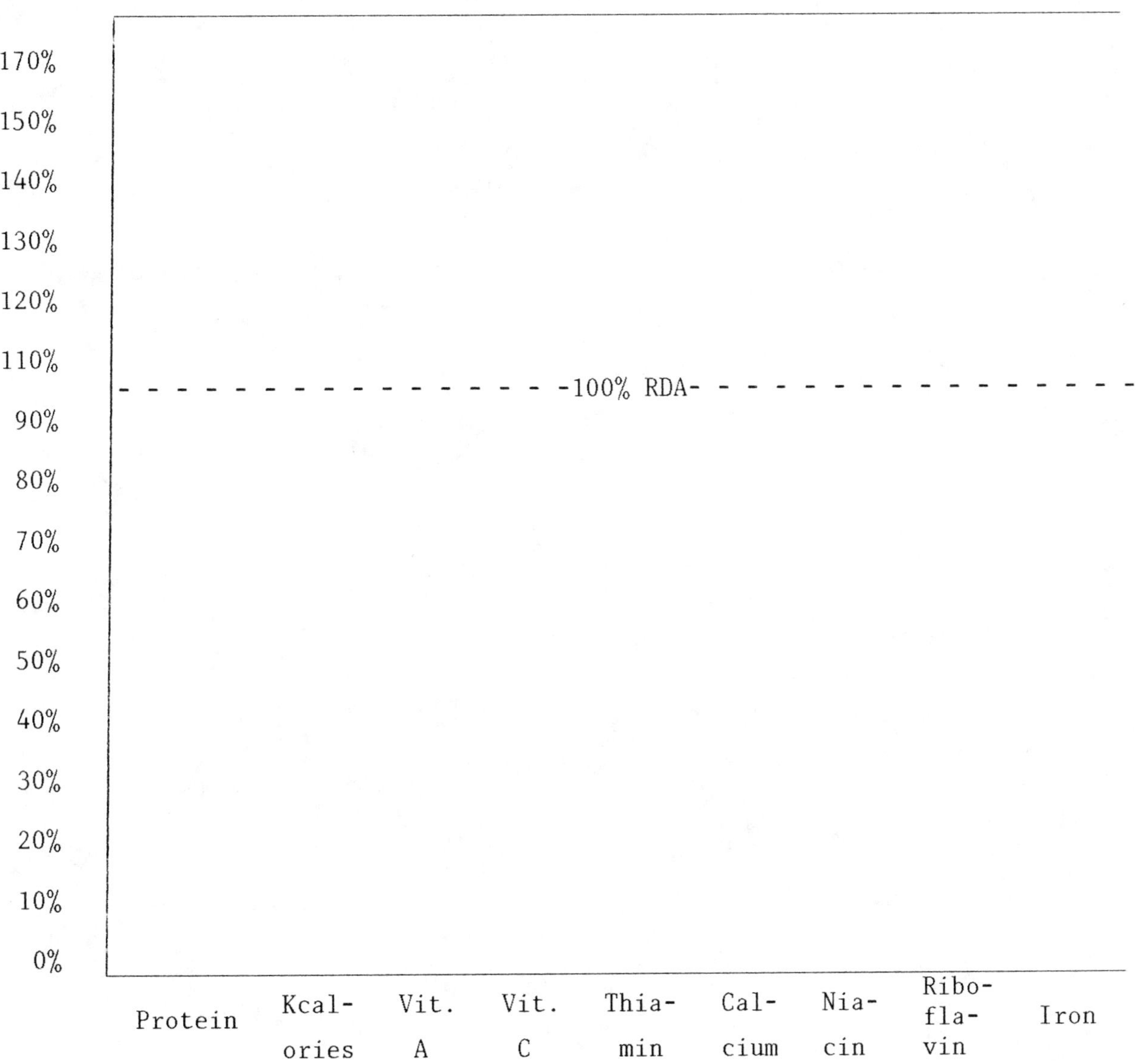

Study Questions:

1. What changes, if any, should you make in your food intake?

2. Discuss the nutrients and any changes needed.

   a. How do your percentages of calories from protein, carbohydrate and fat compare to the American diet?

   b. Compare the amount of protein from animal and plant sources.

   c. Discuss nutrients that exceed the RDA and nutrients that are below two-thirds the RDA.

3. Discuss any supplements being taken. Are they necessary?

4. How does the average American weight compare with the "ideal"? Are American, and you, underweight, overweight, underfat or overfat? Explain. How can your values for fat and muscle stores be altered?

5. Discuss any possible problems of studying undernutrition and overnutrition from your nutritional assessment profile.

References

Acheson, K.J., I.T. Campbell, O.G. Edholm, D.S. Miller and M.J. Stock: The measurement of food and energy intake in man - An evaluation of some techniques. American Journal of Clinical Nutrition. 33: 1147, 1980.

Balogh, M., H.A. Kahn, and J. Medalie: Random repeat 24-Hour dietary recalls. American Journal of Clinical Nutrition, 24; 304, 1974.

Evans, H.K. and D.J. Gines: Dietary recall method comparison for hospitalized elderly subjects. Journal of the American Dietetic Association, 85: 202, 1985.

Jackson, A.S. and M.L. Pollock: Practical assessment of body composition. The Physician and Sports Medicine, 13: 76, 1985.

Bishop, C.W.: Norms for nutritional assessment of American adults by upper arm circumference. American Journal of Clinical Nutrition, 34(11): 2540, 1981.

Keys, A.F. and Fidanza, M.J. et al.: Indicies of relative weight and obesity. Journal of Chronic Disease, 25: 329, 1972.

Marjonnier, L., and Y. Hall: The National Diet Heart Study, assessment of dietary adhearance. Journal of the American Dietetic Association, 52: 288, 1968.

Murray, R.: Discussion and critique of current methods in anthropometry, Part I. Nutrition Support Services, 1: 31, 1981.

Murray, R.: Discussion of techniques in anthropometry, Part II. Nutrition Support Services, 2: 11, 1982.

Pao, E.M., S.J. Mickles, and M.C. Burke: One-day and 3-day nutrient intakes by individuals -- nationwide food consumption survey findings, Spring 1977. Journal of American Dietetic Association, 85: 313, 1985.

Shanklin, D., J.M. Endres, and M. Sawicki: A comparative study of two nutrient data bases. Journal of the American Dietetic Association, 85: 308, 1985.

Swan, P.B.: Food consumption by individuals in the United States: Two major surveys. Annual Review of Nutrition, 3: 413, 1983.

Toledo Dietetic Association. Toledo Diet Manual. Toledo, Ohio, 1982.

Reshef, A., and L. Epstein: Reliability of a dietary questionnaire. American Journal of Clinical Nutrition, 25: 91, 1972.

West, K.M.: Computing and expressing degrees of fatness (letter to the editor). Journal of the American Medical Association, 243: 1421, 1980.

LESSON 2

Labeling and the USRDA

Objectives:

At the conclusion of this lesson, the student will be able to:

- Explain the difference between the RDA and USRDA.
- List the information that is mandatory on the food labels.
- List three optional ingredients on a food label.
- Use nutrition labeling correctly to compare nutrient content of foods.

Equipment:

Frozen or canned food labels or access to a grocery store:
- Broccoli
- Green Beans
- Peas
- Corn
- Mixed Vegetables

USRDA Chart

Procedure:

Compare the nutrient content and cost of different vegetables by using nutrition labeling in the following way:

1. On Table 7, use the food labels from the vegetables. Use the same brand and size package, if possible.
2. Write down the net weight of each container on the chart. Write down the total cost of each container.
3. Write down the serving size, as listed on the nutritional labeling.
4. Fill in the number of servings per package (as listed on the label) on the chart.
5. Using the nutrition labeling, write the percentage of the USRDA for Vitamin A that is supplied by one serving of the vegetable.
6. Repeat Step 5, finding the value for Vitamin C.

Table 7.

Comparison of Nutrient Content

Information	Broccoli	Green Beans	Peas	Corn	Mixed Vegetables (frozen)
Brand Name					
Net Weight of package					
Cost of package					
Serving Size					
Servings per container					
% of USRDA in 1 serving/A					
% of USRDA in 1 serving/C					
Adult USRDA for Vit. A					
I.U. Vit. A per serving					
Cost per serving					

Evaluation:

1. On the USRDA chart, find the adult value for Vitamin A. Write this on the chart under each vegetable.

2. Next, find the I.U. of Vitamin A supplied by one serving of the vegetable in the following way:

   Multiply the I.U. of Vitamin A in the USRDA by the percent supplied by one vegetable serving.

   Example:

5,000	units Vitamin A
x .02	(2%) percent of USRDA in one serving
100.00	

   There are 100 I.U. of Vitamin A supplied in one serving.

3. Divide the cost of the product package by the number of servings in each package.

   Example: $1.00 divided by 4 servings = $0.25 per serving

Equipment:

Food labels or access to a grocery store:
- Regular canned peas
- Dietetic canned peas
- "Dietetic cookies"
- Low sodium soup
- Dietetic product containing cholestrol content
- Comparable regular product containing nutritional labeling

Procedures:

1. Locate the food items in a grocery store or use package labels provided to you.

2. For the product that contains the cholestrol content, some food items to use might include diet margarine, noodles, or soup.

3. Fill in the proper information on the comparison chart by using the nutritional labeling (Table 8).

4. Write in the brand name of the products used. Specify the cholesterol product you are going to use.

5. Fill in the weight of the cans or packages.

6. Fill in the price of each package.

7. Fill in the size of a single serving according to the nutritional labeling.

8. Fill in the number of servings per container, according to the nutritional labeling.

9. Fill in the grams of carbohydrate per serving.

10. Fill in the grams of fat per serving, as stated on the nutrition label.

11. Write in any optional ingredients that are listed on the label.

12. Fill in the amount of the optional ingredients.

    Example: Cholesterol: 9 mg/100 g
    10 g

Evaluation:

1. Determine the cost per serving of each food item. Divid the total cost of the package by the number of servings on the package.

    Example: $0.25 divided by 5 servings = $0.05 per serving

Table 8.

Optional Nutrients

Item	Regular Canned Peas	Dietetic Soup/Peas	Low Sodium Soup	Diet Cookies	Chol. Restric. Food	Regular Chol. Food
Brand Name						
Package size						
Package Cost						
Serving Size						
Servings/ container						
Cal./Serv.						
CHO/Serv. (g)						
Fat/Serv. (g)						
Optional Nutrients Listed on Label						
Amount of Optional Nutrients						
Cost per serving						

Study Questions:

1. What are the major areas of difference between the 1980 RDA and the USRDA's used on labeling?

2. What is the purpose of nutrition labeling? What are some practical applications for the information found on the nutrition labeling? Why aren't fresh fruits and vegetables required to have nutrition labeling?

3. Name three (3) optional ingredients found on nutrition labeling. What food groups or items are these optional ingredients found on?

4. After reading the nutrition labeling and completing the exercises, decide if diet foods are always lower in calories.

References

A statement by the Food and Nutrition Board: Recommended dietary allowances: Scientific issues and process for the future. Journal of Nutrition Education, 18, 82, 1986.

Cooke, J.R.: Food composition tables -- Analytical problems in the collection of data. Human Nutrition: Applied Nutrition, 37A, 441, 1983.

Dubick, M.A.: Dietary supplements and health aids -- A critical evaluation. Part 2 -- Macronutrients and fiber. Journal of Nutrition Education, 15, 88, 1983.

Food and Nutrition Board: Recommended Dietary Allowances, 9th edition, Washington: National Research Council-National Academy of Sciences, 1980.

Forbes, A.L.: Revision of the Food Label. Cereal Food World, 216: 661, 1981.

Guthrie, J.A.: Selection and quantification of typical food portions by young adults. Journal of the American Dietetic Association, 84, 1440, 1984.

Harper, A.: Nutritional regulations and legislation-post developments, future implications. Journal of the American Dietetic Association, 71: 601, 1977.

Marks, L.: What's in a label? Consumers, public policy and food labels. Food Policy, 9, 252, 1984.

Marshall, E.: The academy kills a nutrition report. Science, 230, 420, 1985.

Morrison, M.: A consumer's guide to food labels. FDA Consumer, 11: No. 5, 1977. HEW Publication No.(FDA) 77-2083.

Nutrition and Your Health, Dietary Guidelines for Americans, 2nd edition, Home and Garden bulletin No. 232, U.S. Department of Agriculture, and Department of Health and Human Services, Washington, D.C., 1985.

Miller, S.A. and Stephenson, M.G.: Scientific and public health rationale for the dietary guidelines for Americans. American Journal of Clinical Nutrition, 42, 739, 1985.

Taylor, D.L.: Regulating the nutrition label: Will lawmakers tighten the reins? Food Engineering, page 19, January 1986.

Wretland, A.: Standards for nutritional adequacy of the diet: European and WHO/FAO viewpoints. American Journal of Clinical Nutrition, 36, 366, 1982.

Zempel, C.: Food Labeling: ADA comments to the Food and Drug Administration. Journal of the American Dietetic Association, 73: 664, 1978.

LESSON 3

Proteins and Amino Acids

Part 1. Protein Content of Foods

Objectives:

Upon completion of the lesson, the student will be able to:

- Evaluate and compare some foods as sources of protein.
- List protein values of various foods.
- Determine ways, means, and ease of obtaining definite amounts of protein in the diet.
- Discuss problems involved in planning for protein adequacy in meatless or low-meat diets.
- Explain the difference between animal and plant protein.

Equipment and Materials:

Food Models (Dairy Council or Nasco)*
USDA Handbooks Nos. 8, 72, 456

Procedure and Evaluation:

1. Use the handbooks to determine the common serving size of the foods assigned to you. Record the common serving size and the number of grams of protein in the food portion on Table 9. Convert the common measure to gram weight by consulting the conversion chart in the Textbook. Record the gram weight on Table 9.

2. Calculate the per cent protein each food contains.

   Example: $\dfrac{\_\_\_\_\_ \text{ grams of protein}}{\_\_\_\_\_ \text{ gram weight of food protein}} \times 100 =$ ____% protein in the food portion

3. Calculate the per cent of the RDA for protein each food portion provides:

   Example: $\dfrac{\_\_\_\_\_ \text{ grams of protein in food portion}}{\_\_\_\_\_ \text{ grams of protein for your RDA}} \times 100 =$ ____% RDA for protein furnished in one food portion

4. Determine the number of servings of each food that would furnish approximately 10 grams of protein. Record on Table 10.

5. Determine the protein category for each food:

Category	Grams of Protein/Serving
Low (L)	0 - 3
Medium (M)	4 - 9
High (H)	10 and over

Complete the Protein Category column on Table 9.

6. Complete a bar graph for each food item on Form 2. Grams of protein per serving should be on the vertical axis with the food items on the horizontal axis.

All the foods considered high in protein should be side by side.
All the foods considered to have medium content should by side by side.
All the foods considered to be low in protein should be side by side.

Note:
1. Cooked food weights are to be used.
*2. Optional Activity: Arrange food models in display areas according to protein content per serving.

Table 9.
Portions of Common Foods Containing the Equivalent of Protein Obtained in One Average Serving of Meat

Food	Serving Portion					Servings Equal to 10 g Protein	Protein L, M, H
	Size or Common Serving	Wt. g	Protein g/serving	% Protein	% RDA		
1. Whole Milk							
2. Buttermilk							
3. Skim Milk							
4. Cheddar Cheese							
5. Cottage Cheese							
6. Ice Cream							
7. Spinach							
8. Carrots							
9. Tomatoes							
10. Broccoli							
11. Cabbage							
12. Corn							
13. Ground Round Steak							
14. Pork Chop							
15. Liver							
16. Lima Beans							
17. Baked Beans							
18. White Bread							
19. Spaghetti							
20. Noodles							
21. Dry Peas							
22. Oatmeal							
23. Corn Flakes							
24. Egg, cooked							

Form 2.

Protein Graph

PERCENT

FOODS

Part 2. Protein Adequacy

1. Plan a two day diet for a non-vegetarian (each day's menu should contain at least 40 grams of protein). Write these menus on Form 3.

   Use only the accepted form for writing menus. Use good style. The menus in both sections will be evaluated for color, flavor, texture, temperature, and the Basic Four. Consider variety in breads and cereals.

2. Complete two days of menus for a partial vegetarian. Complete two days of menus for a pure vegetarian (vegan). Write these menus for Form 4.

3. Select what you consider the best one day's menu for both the vegan and the partial vegetarian. Record the foods from these menus on Table 10 & 11. Use handbooks 8, 72, or 456 to determine the grams of protein in each item. Record this on the tables. Figure the per cent protein and the per cent of the RDA for protein that each food provides. Determine if the biological value is high, medium or low and record this on the table.

Form 3.

Non-Vegetarian Menus

Days	Breakfast	Lunch	Dinner
Day One			
Day Two			

Form 4. (a)

Vegetarian Menus (Day 1)

Type	Breakfast	Lunch	Dinner
Pure Vegetarian (Vegan)			
Partial Vegetarian			

Form 4. (b)

Vegetarian Menus (Day 2)

Type	Breakfast	Lunch	Dinner
A Pure Vegetarian (1)			
Partial Vegetarian (2)			

(1) pure vegetarian: one who consumes only food of plant origin without specific restrictions as to kind.

(2) partial vegetarian: one who consumes foods of plant origin and selected food of animal origin, such as milk (lacto-vegetarian), or eggs (ovo-vegetarian), or both (lacto-ovo-vegetarian).

Table 10.

Protein Supplied From One Day's Diet
(pure vegetarian)

Food	Measure g	Protein g	Per Cent Protein	Per Cent RDA	Biological Value H L

Table 11.

Protein Supplied From One Day's Diet
(partial vegetarian)

Food	Measure g	Protein g	Per Cent Protein	Per Cent RDA	Biological Value H M L

Study Questions:

1. What are the problems in attaining protein adequacy when meat is omitted from the diet?

2. From the list of 24 foods on Table 9, identify all that supply satisfactory levels of essential amino acids. (Refer to p. 54 and pp. 665-669 in Pennington and Church, Food Values of Portions Commonly Used," J.B. Lippincott, 1980).

3. In terms of amino acids, explain the difference between foods said to have high biological value and those having low biological value.

4. Why is it important that all the essential amino acids be included in the diet in adequate amounts in each meal throughout the day?

References

Ballentine, C.: The essential guide to amino acids. FDA Consumer, page 23, September 1985.

Bender, A.E.: Health or Hoax? The Truth About Health Food and Diets. Elvendon Press, Goring-on-Thames, England, page 37, 1985.

Chapra, J.C., A. Forbes, and J. Habicht: Protein in the U.S. Diet. Journal of the American Dietetic Association, 72: 253, 1978.

DiGiovanna, J.J. and Blank, H.: Failure of lysine in frequently recurrent herpes simplex infection. Archives of Dermatology, 120, 48, 1984.

Dwyer, J.T., W.H. Dietz, E.M. Andrew, and R.M. Suskind: Nutritional status of vegetarian children. American Journal of Clinical Nutrition, 35: 204, 1982.

Garza, C., N. Scrimshaw, and V. Young: Human protein requirements: The effect of variations in energy intake within the maintenance range. American Journal of Clinical Nutrition, 29: 280, 1976.

Harper, A.E., P. Payne, and J. Waterlow: Assessment of human protein needs. American Journal of Clinical Nutrition, 26: 1168, 1973.

Irwin, M., and P.M. Hegsted: A Conspectus of Research on Amino Acid Requirements of Man. Journal of Nutrition, 101: 539, 1971.

Iyengar, A.K. and B.S. Narasinga Rao: Effect of varying energy and protein intakes on some biochemical parameters of protein metabolism. American Journal of Clinical Nutrition, 35(4): 733, 1982.

Marsh, A.G., T.V. Sanchez, F.L. Chaffee, G.H. Mayor, and O. Michelsen: Bone mineral mass in adult lacto-ovo-vegetarian and omnivorous males. The Journal of Clinical Nutrition, 37: 453: 1983.

Register, U.D., and L. Sonnenberg: The vegetarian diet. Scientific and practical considerations. Journal of the American Dietetic Association, 62: 253, 1973.

Rennie, M.J. and Harrison, R.: Effects of injury, disease, and malnutrition on protein metabolism in man. Unanswered questions. Lancet, i, 323, 1984.

Summary: Diet and behavior symposium proceedings. Nutrition Reviews, 44, 252, Supplement, May 1986.

Taber, L., and R. Cook: Dietary and anthropometric assessment of adult omnivores, fish eaters, and lacto-ovo-vegetarian. Journal of the American Dietetic Association, 76: 21, 1980.

Wurtman, R.J.: Ways that foods affect the brain. Nutrition Reviews, 44, 2, Supplement, May 1986.

Zidenberg-Cherr, S. and others: Dietary superoxide dismutase does not affect tissue levels. American Journal of Clinical Nutrition, 37, 5, 1983.

LESSON 4

Carbohydrate and Fiber

Objectives:

At the conclusion of this lesson, the student will be able to:

- Identify the food groups which are highest in fiber.
- Identify the food groups that contain the highest percentage of carbohydrate.
- Determine the percent of calories in a diet that are derived from carbohydrate.

Materials and Equipment:

Pennington and Church, Food Values of Portions Commonly Used, J.B. Lippincott, 1980.
USDA Handbook Nos. 8-1 through 8-9, 72, 456.
Fast Food Reference List (Ross Laboratories)
Exchange Lists for Meal Planning (Refer to the Textbook in Robinson & Lowler, Normal and Therapeutic Nutrition, 16th ed., MacMillan, 1982, p. 660, Table A-4)

Procedure and Evaluation:

Part 1.

1. Using Table 12 and Handbook 8, 72 or 456, find out the grams in a single serving of the foods listed. Record on Table 12.

2. Using the handbooks, record the carbohydrate content in grams. Record the calorie content also.

3. Next, find the crude fiber content and record. Use Pennington and Church and USDA Handbook No. 8 as the reference for this.

4. Finally, determine the percent of carbohydrate each food contains in the following way:

$$\frac{\text{grams of CHO}}{\text{grams of food item}} \times 100 = \_\_\_\_\% \text{ Carbohydrate}$$

Table 12.
Relative Carbohydrate Content

Food	Single Serving Common Weight	Weight (g)	Calories	Carbo-hydrate (g)	Fiber	% CHO
1. Orange juice						
2. Fresh orange						
3. Fresh apple						
4. Skim Milk						
5. Baked potato						
6. Big Mac						
7. Pork chop (2 oz.)						
8. Soft drink						
9. Whole milk						
10. White bread						
11. Whole wheat bread						
12. Liver (2 oz.)						
13. Raw carrots						
14. Cooked carrots						
15. Cornflakes						
16. French fries						
17. All Bran						
18. Raisin Bran						
19. Lettuce						
20. Cabbage						
21. Pizza, cheese (1 slice)						
22. Chocolate bar						
23. Apple pie						
24. Ice cream						

Part 2.

1. On Table 13, record the food items you consumed in the first day of your dietary intake. Copy the weight in grams and the caloric content.

2. Record the carbohydrate content.

3. Next, determine the carbohydrate content by the exchange group method. Using the Exchange Lists (Diabetic) that is in your textbook, record the carbohydrate content of each item.

4. Determine the total amount of calories in your diet derived from carbohydrate.

   Add up all the grams of carbohydrate.
   Multiply by 4 to determine the number of calories from CHO.

   Example:

200	g CHO
x 4	calories per gram CHO
800	calories from CHO

   Do this using the carbohydrate content that was found using the handbooks, and also using the exchange method.

5. Determine the percent of calories derived from CHO that you consumed.

   Example: $\frac{\text{calories from CHO}}{\text{total calories}} \times 100 = \_\_\_\_\_\%$ calories from CHO

6. Determine the fiber content of each food item, using Bowes and Church. Record. Total the amount of fiber and record.

7. Complete the study questions. Complete a generalization on the lab.

Table 13.

Carbohydrate and Fiber Content of Diet

Food	Weight (g)	Calories	CHO by Handbook	CHO Exchange Method[a]	Crude Fiber
Total					

Calories from CHO _____

Per cent of calories from CHO _____

a. Refer to the textbook.

Study Questions:

1. How did the method of calculation affect the carbohydrate value of your diet study? Which method (the Handbook, or the Exchange System) was most accurate? Which method was faster? Which method was most practical for casual use? Which method is most applicable for intake studies?

2. What food or food groups contain the most fiber? Are some "high fiber" foods misleading? Is there a significant difference between the fiber content of white and whole wheat bread?

3. Do you believe the carbohydrate content of your diet should be raised or lowered? What changes would you make in your diet to accomplish this?

4. Correct the following misconceptions concerning carbohydrate content and fiber:

   Potatoes are really starchy and full of calories.
   Foods that are 100% carbohydrate are always high in calories.
   Fast food items are mainly just starch.
   You shouldn't eat white bread since it has no fiber and has a lot of calories in it.

References

Barry, H.M.: Addressing confusion over the role of modified starches. Food Engineering, page 56, January 1986.

Bing, F.C.: Dietary fiber - in historical perspective. Journal of the American Dietetic Association 69: 498, 1976.

Bolton, R.P., K.W. Heaton, and L.F. Burroughs: The role of dietary fiber in satiety, glucose and insulin: Studies with fruit and fruit juice. The American Journal of Clinical Nutrition, 34(2): 211, 1981.

Burkitt, D.P. and others: Prevalence of diverticular disease, hiatus hernia, and pelvic phleboliths in black and white Americans. Lancet, ii, 880, 1985.

Gray, G.E.: Diet, crime and delinquency: A critique. Nutrition Reviews, 44 (Supplement), 89, 1986.

Groothuis, J.R. and others: Effect of carbohydrate ingested on outcome in infants with mild gastroenteritis. Journal of Pediatrics, 108, 903, 1986.

Henry, R.R. and others: Metabolic consequences of very-low-calorie diet therapy in obese non-insulin-dependent diabetic and nondiabetic subjects. Diabetes, 35, 155, 1986.

Kelsay, J.L.: A Review of Research on Effects of Fiber Intake on Man. American Journal of Clinical Nutrition, 31: 142, 1978.

Lanza, E. and Butrum, R.R.: A critical review of food fiber analysis and data. Journal of the American Dietetic Association, 86, 731, 1986.

Marlett, J.A., and R.L. Bokram: Relationship between calculated dietary and crude fiber intakes of 200 college students. American Journal of Clinical Nutrition, 34(3): 335, 1981.

Morgan, K.J. and M.E. Zabik: Amount and food sources of total sugar intake by children ages 5 to 12 years. American Journal of Clinical Nutrition, 34(3): 404, 1981.

Newcomer, A.D. and McGill, D.B.: Clinical importance of lactase deficiency. New England Journal of Medicine, 310, 42, 1984.

Patrow, C.J. and Marlett, J.A.: Variability in the dietary fiber content of wheat and mixed-grain commercial breads. Journal of the American Dietetic Association, 86, 794, 1986.

Van Soest, P.J.: What is fiber and fiber in food. Nutrition Review, 35: 12, 1977.

Walker, A.R.P.: Diet and dental caires: A sceptical view. American Journal of Clinical Nutrition, 43, 969, 1986.

Wilson, D.P. and Endres, R.K.: Compliance with blood glucose monitoring in children with type I diabetes mellitus. Journal of Pediatrics, 108, 1022, 1986.

LESSON 5

Lipids or Fats

Objectives:

At the conclusion of this lesson, the student will be able to:

- Identify food groups that are high or low in cholesterol content.
- Identify food groups that are high or low in total fat content.

Equipment and Materials:

USDA Food Composition Handbooks Nos. 8-1 through 8-6, 72, and 456
Fast Foods Reference List
Feeley, R., Crimer, P.E., and Watt, B. "Cholesterol Content of Foods," *Journal of the American Dietetic Association*, *61*: 134, 1972.

Procedures and Evaluation:

1. Find the common serving size (use 3 ounces for meat portions) for the foods on Table 14. Change the common serving size to grams and record. Look up the cholesterol content and record. Place all the foods into the following groups:

   Low Cholesterol = <20 mg. cholesterol/serving
   Moderate Cholesterol = 20-64 mg. cholesterol/serving
   High Cholesterol = 65 mg. or more cholesterol/serving

2. Using the first day of the dietary intake from Lesson 1: record the foods, the serving size in grams, and the total fat content in grams on Table 16.

3. Find the cholesterol content of each food item and record on Table 16.

4. Find the percent of total fat each food contains in the following way:

$$\frac{\text{g of fat}}{\text{g of total food portion}} \times 100 = \_\_\_\_\%\text{ of fat in food serving}$$

   Record on Table 16. Calculate the total percentage of fat in your day's diet.

5. Calculate the percent of calories derived from fat. Use the following method:

$$\frac{\_\_\_\_\text{ Kcalories of fat/food portion}}{\_\_\_\_\text{ Kcalories (total)/food portion}} \times 100 = \_\_\_\_\%\text{ Kcalories of fat}$$

Table 14.

List of Foods

Foods	Serving Size	Gram	Cholesterol (mg)
1. Cheddar Cheese			
2. Whole Milk			
3. Apple			
4. Baked Potato			
5. McDonald's French Fries			
6. 2% Fat Milk			
7. Corn Flakes			
8. Peas			
9. Sausage			
10. Skim Milk			
11. Tuna			
12. Chicken			
13. Egg, Whole			
14. White Bread			
15. Hog Dog			
16. Green Beans			
17. Pork Loin			
18. Beef, Roast			
19. Big Mac			
20. Liver			
21. Margarine			
22. Butter			
23. Mayonnaise			
24. Lettuce			

Table 15.

Relative Cholesterol Content

Level of Food	Foods	Common Serving Size	g	Cholesterol (mg)
High				
Medium				
Low				

Table 16.

Cholesterol and Fat Content of Diet

Foods	Servings (g)	Total Fat (g)	Choles-terol (mg)	% Fat	% of KCalories from Fat per Food Portion	KCalorie (total) Food Portion
TOTAL						

Study Questions:

1. Identify major groups of foods that are extremely high and low in cholesterol. Do the same for the fat content.

2. Would a diet low in cholesterol also be low in fat? Explain.

3. Does your fat intake account for more than 40% of your total caloric intake? If so, name some practical ways of lowering your intake.

4. The American Heart Association suggests that Americans keep their cholesterol intake below 600 mg. and, perferably, to 300 mg. or lower. Does your diet meet this standard? If not, what could you change to comply with this recommendation?

5. What are some of the factors that affect the amount and type of fat Americans (and you, in particular) eat?

References

Dietary fat and cancer: Specific action or caloric effect? Carroll, K.K. and Reddy, B.S.: _Journal of Nutrition_, _116_, 1130 and 1132, 1986.

Flynn, M.A., B. Heine, G.B. Nolph, H.D. Naumann, E. Parisi, D. Ball, G. Krause, M. Ellersieck and S.S. Ward: Serum lipids in humans fed diets containing beef or fish and poultry. _The American Journal of Clinical Nutrition_, _34_(12): 2734, 1981.

Flynn, M.A., H.D. Naumann, G.B. Nolph, G. Krause, and M. Ellersieck. "Dietary 'meats' and serum lipids," _American Journal of Clinical Nutrition_, _35_(5): 935, 1982.

Greenwald, P. and others: Diet and chemoprevention in NCI's research strategy to achieve national cancer control objectives. _Annual Review of Public Health_, _7_, 267, 1986.

Grundy, S.M.: Comparison of monounsaturated fatty acids and carbohydrates for lowering plasma cholesterol. _New England Journal of Medicine_, 745, 1986.

Harris, W.S.: Health effects of omega-3 fatty acids. _Contemporary Nutrition_, _10_, No. 8, August, 1985.

Hoeg, J.M. and others: An approach to the management of hyperlipoproteinemia. _Journal of the American Medical Association_, _255_, 512, 1986.

Jukes, T.H., Mayer, J. and Mattson, F.H.: Heated fat. _Journal of the American Medical Association_, _255_, 2080, 1986.

Kay, R.M., Z.I. Sabry, and A. Csima: Multivariate analysis of diet and serum lipids in normal men. _The American Journal of Clinical Nutrition_, _33_, 2566, 1980.

Kromhout, D., Bosschieter, E.B., and Coulander, C. d'L.: The inverse relation between fish consumption and 20-year mortality from coronary heart disease. _New England Journal of Medicine_, _312_, 1205, 1985.

Marshall, W.J. and Ballantyne, F.C.: Current clinical laboratory practice: Investigation of plasma lipids -- which tests and when? _British Medical Journal_, _292_, 1652, 1986.

Mondeika, T.: Cholesterol content of shellfish. _Journal of the American Medical Association_, _254_, 2970, 1985.

O'Connor, T.P. and others: Effect of dietary intake of fish oil and fish protein on the development of L-azaserine-induced preneoplastic lesions in the rat pancreas. _Journal of the National Cancer Institute_, _75_, 959, 1985.

Sinclair, H.M.: Essential fatty acids in perspective. _Human Nutrition: Clinical Nutrition_, _38C_, 245, 1984.

LESSON 6

Energy Expenditure and BMR

Objectives:

Upon completion of the lesson, the student will be able to:

- List the three major factors contributing to the total caloric needs of individuals.
- Identify the effects of each of the three factors that contribute to the total caloric needs.
- Compare Kcalorie expenditures for the various activities in which students engage.
- Estimate personal energy needs for basal metabolism (BMR).
- Discuss laboratory techniques which are available for measuring the resting metabolic rate (rate of heat production) by indirect methods.

Equipment and Materials:

Calculator

Introduction:

Laboratory techniques are available for measuring the total metabolic rate (or rate of heat production) by both direct and indirect methods. These techniques are called:

(1) Direct Calorimetry This involved placing the individuals in a special chamber called a calorimeter and measuring the total amount of heat given off. The metabolic rate can then be calculated from the amount of heat that is given off.

(2) Indirect Calorimetry This involves the calculation of the metabolic rate on the basis of the amount of oxygen consumed and of the carbon dioxide excreted in a given period of time. Since the exchange of these gases is directly proportional to the amount of heat being produced, this provides a simple method for calculating the metabolic rate. A respiratory device attached to the nose is used to determine the oxygen and carbon dioxide content of the inspired and expired air.

Total metabolic rate and, therefore, caloric requirements, are a composite of the calories necessary to support (1) basal metabolism, (2) muscle activity, and (3) the effect of food intake.

Total Metabolic Rate

The three major factors that contribute to the total metabolic rate are illustrated below:

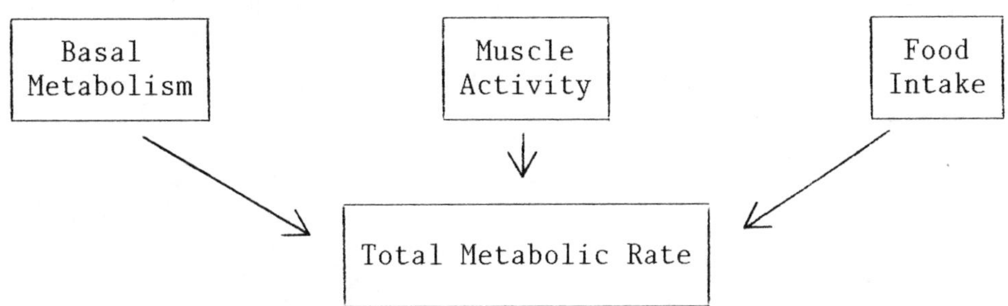

Procedure and Evaluation:

1. Calculation of Basal Metabolism: There are several ways to determine Basal Metabolism.

   (a) Factorial Method. estimate your BMR using the following formula.
   1 Kcalorie per Kg of body weight
   (wt. in Kg = wt. in pounds ÷ 2.2)
   1 Kcal x Kg body wt. x 24 hr. = Kcal (BMR/day)
   1 Kcal/Kg is factor used for men; 0.91 Kcal/Kg is factor used for women.

   (b) Calculate by use of the Harris-Benedict formula.
   Formula for women: $H = 655.0 + 9.6W + 1.9H - 4.7A$
   Formula for men: $H = 66.5 + 13.8W + 5.0H - 6.8A$

   When H = total heat production in 24 hours
   W = body weight in Kg
   H = height in centimeters
   A = age in years

   (c) Calculate by use of a simple formula:
   Actual weight in kilograms x 25 cal/kg
   Where actual weight equals 70 kilograms
   x 25 calories
   1750 calories per 70 kg.

3. Calculate BMRs using the above three methods and record on Table 17.

4. Multiply each BMR figure by 1.3 to estimate total caloric need per day to maintain your actual weight. (This figure assumes you are a person with "average" exercise or muscle activity.) Record on Table 17.

Table 17.

Basal Metabolic Rate

Height	__________ inches		__________ centimeters	
Weight	__________ pounds		__________ kilograms	
Normal weight for age/height/sex __________				
Deviation from "Ideal" weight __________				
BMR:		BMR		Total Calorie Need (BMR x 1.3)
by the factoral methods		______ Kcal		______ Kcal
by the Harris-Benedict formula		______ Kcal		______ Kcal
by a simple formula		______ Kcal		______ Kcal
Average value of the BMR over the 3 methods is			_______ Kcal	
Average total caloric need to maintain weight			_______ Kcal	

3. Determine energy cost of daily physical activity.

(a) For Table 18:

(1) Select one weekday for the 24-hour period. Record date.

(2) Keep a minute-to-minute record of all activity for 24 hours using space provided. Use back for additional space.

(3) Record total number of minutes in last column.

(b) For Table 19:

(1) Summarize your list of activities to those listed on Table 7-2, page 123, in Normal and Therapeutic Nutrition by Robinson and Lowler. List your additional activities in the space provided.

(2) Record total number of minutes for each activity.

(3) Convert minutes to hours. Compare these totals to the ones listed in Table 18 to check accuracy. (Make sure your totals equal to 1440 minutes and 24 hours.)

(c) For Table 20:

(1) Column 1, transfer "time in hours" (last column, Table 19) to "time spent avg./day in hours" (first column, Table 20).

(2) Column 2, using Tables as indicated in Table 20.

(3) Column 3, Column 1 X Column 2.

(4) Column 4, Column 3 X Your Weight in Kg.

(5) Record totals for Columns 1 and 4.

(d) Calculate your total caloric allowances according to the RDA (1980).

Table 18.

Daily Activity Record

Date:

Activity	Time in Minutes		
	Beginning	Ending	Total

Table 19.

Summary of Time Spent in Different Activities

Activity	Time in minutes	Time in hours
	1 Day	1 Day
Dressing, Undressing		
Driving Car		
Eating		
Lying still, awake		
Sitting		
Standing		
Sleeping		
Walking at 3 mph		
Walking down stairs		
Walking up stairs		
Writing		
Total		
Your total should equal	1440	24

Table 20.

Summary of One Day's Energy Expenditure for Activities

Activity (Add others as needed)	Time Spent Avg./day in hours	Kcal/lb./hr.* or Kcal/kg./hr.	Column I x Column II	Kcal/Individual Col. III x your wt. in kg.
Dressing				
Driving Car				
Eating				
Lying still, awake				
Sitting				
Sleeping				
Standing				
Walking at 3 mph				
Walking up stairs				
Writing				
Total				

*See Tables, and Data available in Guthrie, Introductory Nutrition, 5th ed., St. Louis: Mosby, 1983, p. 111; and Briggs and Calloway, Bogart's Nutrition and Physical Fitness, 10th ed., Philadelphia: Saunders Co., 1979, pp. 40-45.

Study Questions:

1. What is the best guide for determining adequacy of caloric intake for an individual?

2. Indicate the influence of the following factors on the basal metabolic rate my marking (↑) next to those factors tending to increase basal metabolism and (↓) next to those factors tending to decrease basal metabolism.

_____ Increased thyroid gland activity
_____ Sleep
_____ Underweight
_____ Fear and anger
_____ Anger
_____ Preschool (very young) Children
_____ Large Skin Surface Area
_____ Pregnancy and Lactation
_____ Elevated Body Temperature
_____ Cold Climate
_____ Elderly Person

Would males or females tend to have a higher metabolic rate? Why?

3. How did you calculated energy expenditure (using your activity record) differ from your BMR and total caloric need estimates? Why?

4. Adjust your recommended caloric need to a diet that would allow you to gain one pound per week; also to a weight reduction diet that would allow you to lose one pound per week. Plan one day's menu for each.

References

Belko, A.Z. and others: Effect of energy and protein intake and exercise intensity on the thermic effect of food. American Journal of Clinical Nutrition, 43, 863, 1986.

Himms-Hagen, J.: Brown adipose tissue metabolism and thermogenesis. Annual Review of Nutrition, 5, 69, 1985.

Jhangiani, S.S. and others: Energy expenditure in chronic alcoholics with and without liver disease. American Journal of Clinical Nutrition, 44, 323, 1986.

Jacobs, M.B. and Wilson, W.: Iron deficiency anemia in a vegetarian runner. Journal of the American Medical Association, 252, 481, 1984.

Kris-Etherton, P.M.: Nutrition and the exercising female. Nutrition Today, page 6, March/April 1986.

Koivisto, V.A.: The physiology of marathon running. Science Progress, 70, 109, 1986.

Lehtonen, A. and Viikari, J.: Serum lipids in soccer and ice-hockey players. Metabolism, 29, 36, 1980.

Owen, O.E. and others: A reappraisal of caloric requirements in healthy women. American Journal of Clinical Nutrition, 44, 1, 1986.

Slavin, J.L. and Joensen, D.J.: Caffeine and sports performance. The Physician and Sport Medicine, page 191, May 1985.

Webb, P.: 24-hour energy expenditure and menstrual cycle. American Journal of Clinical Nutrition, 44, 614, 1986.

LESSON 7

Nutrient Density

Objectives:

At the conclusion of this lesson, the student will be able to:

- Identify relative Kcaloric values of foods.
- Illustrate the concept of Index of Nutritional Quality (INQ).
- Apply the concept of the nutrient density in a food selection.
- Use the concept of the nutrient density as a teaching tool.

Equipment and Materials:

Balance Scale and Weights
Plastic Wrap
Food Items - one per person
Handbooks Nos. 8, 72, 456

Procedures and Evaluation:

A. Index of Nutritional Quality (INQ) - Nutrient density or INQ refers to the amount of nutrients in relation to the amount of kilocalorie in a food. The nutrient density of a serving of food can be determined by calculating its index of nutritional quality (INQ).

To find INQ for a particular nutrient in a given food, there are two basic equations necessary in calculating the INQ value:

(I)

$$\text{\% Standard (\% RDA OR \% USRDA)} = \frac{\text{amount of nutrient in food}}{\text{RDA (or USRDA) for nutrient}} \times 100$$

(II)

$$\text{INQ} = \frac{\text{\% standard for nutrient}}{\text{\% standard for energy}}$$

The nutrient standard can be the RDA for a specific age or sex group or its USRDA.

1. Determine the amount of nutrient and energy for protein, calcium, sodium, iron, Vitamin A, and Ascorbic acid of the food items assigned to you.

2. Next, find out the % Standard for nutrient and the % Standard for energy of each food by using equation I.

3. By using these two standards, compute the Index for Nutritional Quality value for the nutrient in a food.

   Example: Use an orange (medium) as an example to calculate INQ for Vitamin C for a five-year-old boy. RDA for Vitamin C for the boy is 45 mg. RDA for energy for the boy is 1700 Kcal. Vitamin C in one medium size orange is 66 mg. Energy value in one medium size orange is 65 Kcal.

$$\underset{(144)}{\%\ \text{Standard for}}\ \underset{(\text{Vit. C})}{\text{Nutrient}} = \frac{65\ \text{mg}}{45\ \text{mg}} \times 100$$

$$\underset{(3.8)}{\%\ \text{Standard for Energy}} = \frac{65\ \text{Kcal}}{1700\ \text{Kcal}} \times 100$$

$$\text{INQ for Vitamin C} = \frac{\%\ 144\ \text{of Vit. C Std.}}{\%\ 3.8\ \text{of Energy Std.}}$$

INQ = 37.8

* This is the INQ value for Vitamin C in an average orange.

4. Complete Table 21.

5. Answer the study questions.

B. Energy Density (Kaloric)

1. Determine the gram weight and the Kcalorie content of an average serving of the food item(s) assigned to you. Next, find out the gram weight of a 100 Kcalorie portion by setting up a proportion similar to the following example:

   Example: Roast Beef 84 grams = 225 Kcalories

$$\text{Proportion:} \quad \frac{84\ \text{grams}}{225\ \text{Kcalories}}\ \text{is to}\ \frac{X}{100\ \text{Kcalories}}$$

$$8400\ \text{gm/Kcal} = 225\ X\ \text{Kcal}$$
$$X = 37\ \text{grams}$$
$$37\ \text{grams} = 100\ \text{Kcalories}$$

2. Weigh out the 100 Kcal. portions of your assigned food(s). Protect the scale with plastic wrap.

3. Arrange the food in the display area in the order of their weight.
4. Determine the number of servings each 100 Kcalorie portion represents.
5. Complete Tables 21 and 22.
6. Answer the study questions.

Table 21.

Index of Nutritional Quality (INQ)

Food / Food Population	Nutrient	% Standard for Nutrient	% Standard for Energy	INQ	Rank
(1) Baked Potato (Med) for infant (5 months old)	Protein				
	Calcium				
	Iron				
	Vitamin A				
	Vitamin C				
	Sodium				
(2) Milk (8 oz) (skim or whole) pre-school child (3 year old girl)	Protein				
	Calcium				
	Iron				
	Vitamin A				
	Vitamin C				
	Sodium				
(3) Bread (1 slice white) teenager (13 year old boy)	Protein				
	Calcium				
	Iron				
	Vitamin A				
	Vitamin C				
	Sodium				
(4) Coca Cola (8 oz) elderly (70 year old male)	Protein				
	Calcium				
	Iron				
	Vitamin A				
	Vitamin C				
	Sodium				

Table 22.

Caloric Density

Foods				Weigh in Grams of 100 Kcalories	Number of Servings per 100 Kcalories
	Svg.Size	gm	Kcal		
1. Apple					
2. Applesauce					
3. Cabbage					
4. Margarine					
5. Hamburger					
6. Cooked Boiled Potatoes					
7. Frozen Broccoli (cooked)					
8. Bread					
9. Lettuce					
10. Milk, Skim					
11. Milk, Whole					
12. Potato Chips					
13. Fruit Pie Individual					
14. Corn, Canned or Frozen					
15. Salad Dressing					
16. Rice, Cooked					
17. Cookies					

Study Questions:

1. What is the caloric density of fresh fruits and vegetables as compared to cooked fruits and vegetables?

2. Which foods are lowest in caloric density? Which foods are highest?

3. What effect does the fat content of a food have on caloric density? How does the water content of a food affect its caloric density?

4. Calculate the index of nutritional quality for the nutrients listed in Table A-1 (in your text) for Tomato Juice (6 oz.). Use base of 2000 Kcal and the USRDA (your text p. 325).

5. Two teenagers (a boy and a girl) had hot dogs for their lunch. Each raw hot dog weighed 2 ounces. One teenager received more Kcalories in her hot dog than did the other. Discuss.

References

Acheson, K.J., I.T. Campbell, O.G. Edholm, D.S. Miller, and M.J. Stock: The measurement of food and energy intake in man--An evaluation of some techniques. The American Journal of Clinical Nutrition, 33: 1147, 1980.

Bradfield, R.D., editor: Assessment of typical daily energy expenditure. Symposium, American Journal of Clinical Nutrition, 24: 1109, 1971.

Cunningham, J.J.: An individualization of dietary requirements for energy in adults. Journal of the American Dietetic Association, 80: 335, 1980.

Cunningham, J.J.: A reanalysis of factors influencing basal metabolic rate in normal adults. American Journal of Clinical Nutrition, 33: 2372, 1980.

Hansen, R.G., and Wyse, B.W.: Expression of nutrient allowances per 1,000 kilocalories. Journal of the American Dietetic Association, 76: 223, 1980.

Hansen, R.G.: An index of food quality. Nutrition Review, 31: 1, 1973.

Harris, J.A. and Benedict, F.G.: A biometric study of basal metabolism in man. Washington, D.C.: Carnegie Institute, Pub. No. 279, 1954.

Hegsted, D.M.: Energy needs and energy utilization. Nutrition Reviews, 32: 33, 1974.

Jackson, A.S. and Pollock, M.L.: Practical assessment of body composition. The Physicial and Sports Medicine, 13, 76, 1985.

Konishi, F. and S.L. Harrison: Body weight gain equivalents of selected foods. Journal of the American Dietetic Association, 70: 365, 1977.

Levine, A. and J.E. Morley: The shortening pathways to appetite control. Nutrition Today, 18: 1, 8, 1983.

Long, C.L., N. Schaffel, J.W. Geiger, W.R. Schiller, et al.: Metabolic response to injury and illness: Estimation of energy and protein needs from indirect calorimetry and nitrogen balance. Journal of Parenteral and Enteral Nutrition, 3: 452, 1979.

Serog, P., M. Apefelbaum, N. Autissier, F. Baigts, L. Brigant, and A. Ktorza: Effects of slimming and composition of diet on VO_2 and thyroid hormones in healthy subjects. The American Journal of Clinical Nutrition, 35: 24, 1982.

Sukhatme, V. and S. Margen: Autoregulatory homestatic nature of energy balance. The American Journal of Clinical Nutrition, 35: 355, 1982.

Symposium on Energy Balance: American Journal of Clinical Nutrition, 8: 527, 1960.

Wait, B., R. Blair, and L. Roberts: Energy intakes of well-nourished children and adolescents. American Journal of Clinical Nutrition, 22: 1383, 1969.

LESSON 8

Vitamins

Objectives:

At the conclusion of this lesson, the student will be able to:

- Discuss vitamin retention methods of food preparation in rleation to acidity.
- Calculate vitamin content of various food stuffs.

Materials and Equipment:

pH meter
vegetables and fruits as indicated
blender

Procedure and Evaluation:

1. Take half-portions of solid foods listed in Table 23 and liquify in blender. Add water as necessary. Transfer each liquified food item to glass cup or beaker.

2. Measure pH of each food item as directed by instructor. Record results in Table 23.

3. After recording results of all items, add 2 Tablespoons of lemon juice or ascorbic acid to benas, peas, carrots and potatoes.

4. Table pH readings of these foods and record again.

5. Look up vitamin values for foods in Table 2 3(p. 73 in your lab manual) and record.

6. For each vitamin recorded in Table 23 note if stability of each nutrient was stable or unstable (use textbooks). If lemon juice was added, indicate if this was a positive factor for retention of each nutrient (record as + or -).

Table 23.
Vitamin Contents in Vegetables and Fruits

Food	Measure	Vitamin Content		Hydrogen Concentration (pH)		Vitamin A Stable	Vitamin C Stable	Greater Stability With Acid	
		Vitamin A (IU)	Vitamin C (mg)	pH	pH with lemon juice			A	C
Tomato Juice									
Banana									
Orange Juice									
Apple Juice									
Canned Peaches									
Canned Apricots									
Canned Kidney Beans									
Canned or Cooked Carrots									
Canned or Cooked Green Beans									
Canned Peas									
Mashed Potatoes									
Avocado									

Questions:

1. What cooking procedures would result in relatively greater vitamin C retention?

2. Name some ways (minimum of three) of preventing loss of vitamins in food preparation and cooking.

3. What types of food would most likely be cooked with an added acid food? What effect would this have on vitamin retention?

References

Alhadeff, L. and others: Toxic effects of water-soluble vitamins. Nutrition Reviews, 42, 33, 1984.

Anderson, S.H. and others: Adult thiamin requirements and the continuing need to fortify processed cereals. Lancet, ii, 85, 1986.

Bowerman, S. and I. Harrill: Nutrient consumption of individuals taking or not taking nutrient supplements. The Journal of the American Dietetic Association, 83(3): 298, 1983.

Chapkin, R.S., B. Haberstroch, J. Liu, and B. Holub. Effect of vitamin and supplementation on serum and high density lipoprotein - cholesterol in patients on maintenance hemodialysis. The American Journal of Clinical Nutrition, 38: 253, 1983.

Kolata, Gina: Does Vitamin A prevent cancer. Science, 223: 1161, March 16, 1984.

Levine, M.: New concepts in the biology and biochemistry of ascorbic acid. New England Journal of Medicine, 314, 892, 1986.

Mawson, A.R.: Hypervitaminosis A toxicity and gout. Lancet, i, 1181, 1984.

Olson, J.A., D.B. Gunning, and R.A. Tilton: Liver concentration of Vitamin A and carotenoids as a function of age and other parameters of American children who died of various causes. The American Journal of Clinical Nutrition, 39: 903, 1984.

Olson, Robert E.: Vitamin B_6 toxicity: A new megavitamin syndrome. Nutrition Reviews, 42 (Z): 44, 1984.

Snook, Jean, C. London, and J. DeLany: Supplementation frequency and ascorbic acid status in adult males. The American Journal of Clinical Nutrition, 37: 532, 1983.

Sommer, A. and others: Impact of Vitamin A supplementation on childhood mortality. Lancet, i, 1169, 1986.

Staab, D.B., R.E. Hodges, W.K. Metcalf, and J.L. Smith: Relationship between Vitamin A and iron in the liver. Journal of Nutrition, 114, 840, 1984.

Read, Marsha H.: Food supplement usage by the elderly. Journal of the American Dietetic Association, 80: 250, 1982.

Reiter, L.A. and others: Adult thiamin requirements and the continuing need to fortifu processed cereals. Lancet, ii, 85, 1986.

Vitetta, E.S., K.A. Krolick, M. Miuama-Inaba, W. Cushley: Immunotoxins: A new approach to cancer therapy. Science, 219: 644, 1983.

Lesson 9

Minerals

Objectives:

At the conclusion of this lesson, the student will be able to:

- Discuss the relative sources of calcium, iron and sodium in various food groups.
- Discuss how food preparation and cultural patterns affect sodium consumption.

Materials and Equipment:

USDA Handbook, Nos. 8 and 72
USRDA Chart, 1980

Procedures and Evaluation:

1. Look up the mineral values for assigned foods on Table 24. Record.

2. Plan a day's menu that meets the adult RDA for iron and calcium. Plan this menu using only 1 glass of milk. Do not use liver. Complete menu on Form 5.

3. Cook frozen green beans (½ cup portions) with the following amounts of salt in each portion:
   0 salt added
   1/8 teaspoon salt
   1/4 teaspoon salt
   1/2 teaspoon salt
   3/4 teaspoon salt
   1 teaspoon salt

4. Cook canned, drained green beans with the same amounts of sodium as listed above.

5. Taste all beans and record preferences using a 1-6 rating scale for each type (canned and frozen). Record on Table 25. Record in handbook sodium values for 1 portion of green beans (frozen and canned).

6. After recording preferences, record sodium content, 1/4 teaspoon of salt = 575 mg.

Table 24.

Mineral Contents of Selected Foods

Food	House hold	g	Sodium (mg)	Calcium (mg)	Iron (mg)
Rice, cooked	½ C				
All Bran Cereal	½ C				
2 eggs	2				
1 cup Milk	1 c.				
Cottage Cheese	½ c.				
Hamburger	3 oz.				
Sliced Turkey	3 oz.				
Ham	3 oz.				
American Cheese	3 oz.				
Broccoli (fresh)	½ C				
Green Beans (canned)	½ C				
Wheat Bread	1 slc.				
White Bread	1 slc.				
Raisins	¼ C				
Apple (medium)	1				
Orange (medium)	1				
Margarine	1 tsp.				

Form 5.

One Day's Menu for Calcium and Iron Content

	Amounts	Foods Consumed	Fe	Ca
Breakfast				
Lunch				
Dinner				
Snacks				

Table 25.

Sodium Content and Taste Preference

Frozen Beans	Taste Preference (1-6)	Sodium Content per 1/2 C. serving
0 Salt		
1/8 t. salt		
1/4 t. salt		
1/2 t. salt		
3/4 t. salt		
1 t. salt		
Canned Beans		
0 Salt		
1/8 t. salt		
1/4 t. salt		
1/2 t. salt		
3/4 t. salt		
1 t. salt		

Study Questions:

1. What are three causes of nutrient loss in cooked foods?

2. Why do we cook foods? What vitamin and mineral may be lost in cooking?

3. Name some says of preventing the loss of vitamin and mineral when cooking foods.

4. Discuss major sources of sodium in the American diet. What are the reasons one may wish to estimate the sodium in the diet and how can one alter this intake without resorting to purchase of "dietetic items"?

5. It is estimated that iron absorption from the intestinal tract may be only 10%. What factors may decrease or enhance absorption? (Review textbook.)

6. What are the problems associated with increasing calcium in the diet if only 1 glass of milk is consumed per day? How are sodium and iron affected if greater amounts of dairy products such as cheese are used as protein sources?

7. How do cultural food patterns affect preference? Explain fully.

References

Allen, L.: Calcium bioavailability and absorption: A review. The American Journal of Clinical Nutrition, 35: 783, 1982.

Beevers, D.G.: Should recommendations be made to reduce dietary sodium intake? The case for recommendations. Proceedings of the Nutrition Society, 45, 263, 1986.

Bertino, M. and others: Increasing dietary salt alters salt taske preference. Physiology and Behavior, 38, 203, 1986.

Brittin, H.C. and Nossaman, C.E.: Iron content of food cooked in iron utensils. Journal of the American Dietetic Association, 86, 897, 1986.

Clark, L.C. and Combs, Jr., G.F.: Selenium compounds and the prevention of cancer: Research needs and public health implications. Journal of Nutrition, 116, 170, 1986.

Eaton, S.B. and Konner, M.: Paleolithic nutrition. New England Journal of Medicine, 312, 283, 1985.

Gordan, G.S. and Vaughan, C.: Calcium and osteoporosis. Journal of Nutrition, 116, 319, 1986.

Gruchow, H.W. and others: Alcohol, nutrient intake, and hypertension in U.S. adults. Journal of the American Medical Association, 253, 1567, 1985.

Hallberg, L. and L. Rossander: Absorption of iron from western-type lunch and dinner. The American Journal of Clinical Nutrition, 35: 502, 1982.

Hypertension: Is there a place for calcium? Lancet, iI, 359, 1986.

Kramer, A. "Storage Retention of Nutrients," Food Technology, 28: 50, 1974.

Krehl, W., and R. Winters: Effects of cooking methods on retention of vitamins and minerals in vegetables. Journal of the American Dietetic Association, 26: 966, 1950.

Lever, A.F.: Should recommendations be made to reduce socium intake? The case against recommendations. Proceedings of the Nutrition Society, 45, 259, 1986.

Milne, D.B., D. Schnakenberg, H.L. Johnson, and G.L. Kuhl: Trace mineral intake of enlisted military personnel. Journal of the American Dietetic Association, 76: 41, 1980.

Ott, S.: Should women get screening bone mass measurements? Annals of Internal Medicine, 104, 874, 1986.

Preer, J.R. and others: Metals in downtown Washington, D.C. gardens. Biological Trace Element Research, 6, 79, 1984.

Spencer, H. and Kramer, L.: Factors contributing to osteoporosis. Journal of Nutrition, 116, 316, 1096.

LESSON 10

Cultural Food Patterns in the U.S.

Objectives:

At the conclusion of this lab, the student will be able to:

- Calculate the nutrient content of a recipe.
- Compare the nutritional value of typical ethnic dishes.
- Discuss the influence of cultural food patterns on American diets.

Materials and Equipment:

Handbooks Nos. 8 and 72
Pennington, and Church, H. Food Values of Portions Commonly Used, Philadelphia: J.B. Lippincott, 1980.
Recipe Ingredients

Procedures and Evaluation:

1. Prepare the assigned recipe on the following page.
2. For your assigned recipe, list the ingredients on Table 26. Calculate the nutrient values for the recipe. Calculate the nutrient value for one serving of the recipe.
3. Share the nutrient value information for your recipe with the other lab units. Record the information on Table 27. Answer the questions on nutrient content of the recipes.
4. Complete a bar graph in the space provided that compares the protein content of the assigned dishes. Place the food items and their country of origin on the horizontal axis and the amount of protein (grams) on the vertical axis. Complete similar graphs for calories, fat, calcium, iron, and sodium.
5. Answer the study questions.

RECIPES

(1) TACOS (Mexican)
2 Taco Shells, cooked
2 oz. hamburger
1 small tomato
1/2 small onion
1/4 c. American cheese, shredded
1/4 pkg. Taco Seasoning Mix
1/8 head lettuce, chopped

Brown hamburger with seasoning mix. Drain. Chop lettuce, tomato, and onion. Fill Taco shells with hamburger mixture and then add onion, tomato, lettuce and cheese.
Yield: 2 servings

(3) CHEESEBURGERS (American)
2 oz. (slices) American cheese
8 oz. hamburger
2 hamburger buns
1 oz. ketchup
2 T. mustard

Form hamburgers into patties. Pan broil. Place in buns and add condiments.
Yield: 2 servings

(5) CHICKEN CHOP SUEY (Oriental)
1/4 lb. chicken, cup up into cubes
1 cup water
3/4 t. salt
(about 1725 mg. of sodium)
1 T. flour
1/8 c. water
1/4 c. slivered green pepper
1 T. chopped onion
1/4 c. slivered celery
1/2 can bean sprouts
1 T. soy sauce
1 c. long grain rice, cooked

Brown chicken in skillet. Add 1 cup water and salt. Simmer about 30 minutes or until tender. Combine flour and 1/8 c. water. Stir into hot meat. Add green pepper, onion, and celery. Boil 15 minutes. Add bean sprouts and soy sauce. Heat on low for 10 minutes. Serve on rice.
Yield: 2 servings

(2) SPAGHETTI (Italian)
2 oz. bulk sausage or hamburger
2 T. oil
1 t. oregano
1/2 clove garlic
8 oz. spaghetti sauce
1/4 c. onion, chopped
3 oz. spaghetti noodles

Brown sausage and drain. Cook onions in oil with oregano and garlic. Blend into spaghetti sauce and simmer. Cook spaghetti noodles in salted boiling water. Drain. Pour spaghettic sauce over noodles.
Yield: 2 servings

(4) SMORREBORD (Scandinavian)
Open Face Sandwiches
2 slices rye bread
1/2 can sardines
3 oz. cream cheese or ham or liverwurst
red radishes, sliced
1 egg, hard boiled
Optional: green onions or cucumber

Spread bread with softened cream cheese. Arrange other food on bread, leaving sandwiches open faced.
Yield: 2 servings

(6) MEAT WITH OKRA (Greece)
1/4 lb. lamb, diced
1 T. olive oil
1/4 c. onion, diced
1/4 lb. tomatoes, peeled and diced
1/4 c. water
1/4 lb. okra or 1/4 box frozen whole okra, thawed
Salt and pepper to taste
Juice of 1/4 lemon

Saute meat very lightly in butter in heavy skillet. Add onions and continue cooking over medium heat for 15 minutes. Add tomatoes and 2 T. of water. Cover skillet, reduce heat and simmer until meat is tender. Arrange okra on top of meat in rows (first removing cone-shaped tops if fresh okra is used). Add salt and pepper, lemon juice and another 2 T. of water. Cover and cook over medium heat until meat is tender (about 30 minutes).
Yield: 2 servings.

Table 26.

Analysis of Ethnic Dishes
(One Serving)

Ingredients	Measure of Serving	Wt. Gm.	Cal-ories Kcal.	Pro-tein Gm.	Fat Gm.	Carbo-hy-drate Gm.	Ca mg.	Na mg.	Fe mg.	Choles-terol- mg.	Thia-mine mg.	Ribo-flavin mg.	Nia-cin mg.	Ascorbic Acid mg.
TOTALS														
%RDA														

Form 6.

Comparing Nutrient Values

PROTEIN COMPARISON

CALORIE COMPARISON

FAT COMPARISON

CALCIUM COMPARISON

IRON COMPARISON

SODIUM COMPARISON

Table 27.

Ethnic Dish Analysis Summary (For 1 serving)

Recipe	Calories	Protein Gm.	Fat Gm.	Carbo-hydrate Gm.	Ca mg	Na mg	Fe mg	Choles-terol mg	Thiamine mg	Ribo-flavin mg	Niacin mg	Ascorbic Acid mg

Which country produce:

the lowest fat recipe? ______________________

the 2 highest fat recipes? __________ & __________

the highest calorie recipe? ______________________

the lowest calorie recipe? ______________________

the higest sodium recipe? ______________________

Which country produce:

the recipe with the highest protein content? ______________

the highest iron recipe? ______________________

the recipe with the lowest iron content? ______________

the recipe with the higest cholesterol content? ____________

the recipe with the lowest calcium content? ______________

<u>Study Questions</u>:

1. How do the representative ethnic dishes reflect the availability or unavailability of agricultural products in the world area where the dishes originated? How does geography affect what is available?

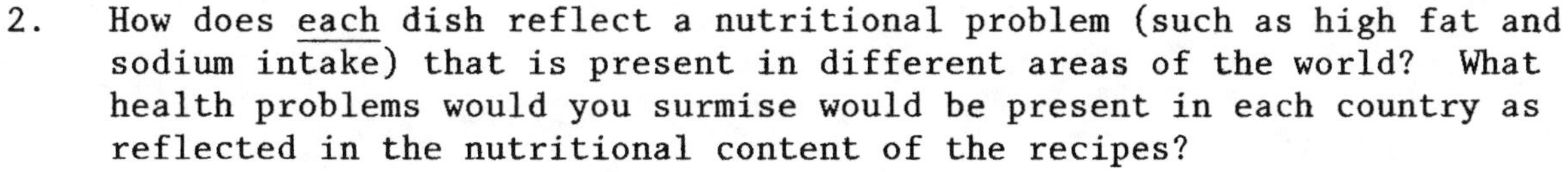

2. How does <u>each</u> dish reflect a nutritional problem (such as high fat and sodium intake) that is present in different areas of the world? What health problems would you surmise would be present in each country as reflected in the nutritional content of the recipes?

3. What are the implications of increasing ethnic dishes into the "typical" American diet? Which nutrients would most likely increase?

4. Are there any ethnic foods in your diet due to the influence of family or friends? What are they? Be specific.

References

Ahrens, E. H. and C.A. Boucher: Composition of a simulated American diet. Journal of the American Dietetic Association, 73: 613, 1978.

Bogert, J., G. Briggs, and D. Calloway: Nutrition and Physical Fitness, 9th edition, Philadelphia: W.B. Saunders Company, 1973.

Bryant, C.A. and others: The Cultural Feast, West Publishing Company, St. Paul, P. 223, 1985; and Lee, W.H., Customers and Pharmacists pay attention to herbs. American Druggist, page 99, February 1986.

Ehnholm, C., J.K. Huttunen, P. Pietnen, U. Leino, M. Mutanen, E. Kostianen, J. Pikkarainen, et al.: Effect of diet on serum lipo proteins in a population with a high risk of coronary heart disease," The New England Journal of Medicine, 307: 850, 1982.

Grivetti, L.E.: Cultural nutrition: Anthropological and geographic themes. Annual Review and Nutrition, 1, 47, 1981.

Holt, B., R.M. Spargo, J.B. Ivenson, G.S. Faulkner, and D.B. Check: Serum and plasma zinc, copper, and iron concentrations in Aboriginal communities of North Western Australia, 33: 119-136, 1980.

Kuhnlein, H.V., D.H. Calloway, and B.F. Harland: Composition of traditional Hopi foods. Journal of the American Dietetic Association, 75: 37, 1979.

Lambert, J.: The effect of urbanization and western foods on infant and maternal nutrition in the South Pacific. Food and Nutrition Bulletin, 4, 11, 1982.

Mitchell, H.S. and S. Santo: Nutritional improvement in Hokkaldo orphanage children, 1960-1970. Journal of the American Dietetic Association, 72: 506, 1978.

Schwerin, H.S., Stanton, J.L., Riley, A.M., et al.: Food eating patterns and health: A reexamination of the Ten State and Hayes I surveys. American Journal of Clinical Nutrition, 34: 568, 1981.

Swan, P.B.: Food consumption by individuals in the United States: Two major surveys. Annual Review of Nutrition, 3, 413, 1983.

Van Staveren, W.A., A.J. Hautvast, M.B. Katan, M.A.J. van Montfort, and H.G.G. van Oostenvan der Goes: Dietary fiber consumption in an adult Dutch population. Journal of the American Dietetic Association, 80: 324, 1982.

Welsh, S.O.: Review of trends in food use in the United States, 1909 to 1980. Journal of the American Dietetic Association, 81(2), 120, 1982.

APPENDICES

Suggested Weights for Heights for Men and Women*

Height (without shoes) inches	Weight (without clothing) Low	Median pounds	High	Height centimeters	Low	Weight Median kilograms	High
Height (without shoes) inches	Weight (without clothing) Low	Median pounds	High	Height centimeters			
Men							
63	118	129	141	160	54	59	64
64	122	133	145	163	55	60	66
65	126	137	149	165	57	62	68
66	130	142	155	167	59	65	70
67	134	147	161	170	61	67	73
68	139	151	166	173	63	69	75
69	143	155	170	175	65	70	77
70	147	159	174	178	67	72	80
71	150	163	178	180	68	74	81
72	154	167	183	183	70	76	83
73	158	171	188	185	72	77	85
74	162	175	192	188	74	80	87
75	165	178	195	191	75	81	89
Women							
60	100	109	118	152	45	50	54
61	104	112	121	155	47	51	55
62	107	115	125	157	49	52	57
63	110	118	128	160	50	54	58
64	113	122	132	163	51	55	60
65	116	125	135	165	53	57	61
66	120	129	139	167	55	59	63
67	123	132	142	170	56	60	65
68	126	136	146	173	57	62	66
69	130	140	151	175	59	64	69
70	133	144	156	178	60	65	71
71	137	148	161	180	62	67	73
72	141	152	166	183	64	69	75

*Data for heights in inches and weights in pounds taken from: Hathaway, M.L. and Foard, E.D. <u>Heights and Weights of Adults in the United States</u>. Home Economics Research Report No. 10, U.S. Department of Agriculture, Washington, D.C., Table 80, p. 111.

Conversions to centimeters and kilograms were rounded off to the nearest whole number.

Average Weights (50th Percentile*) for Women and Men
Aged 18-74 Years in the United States
1971-1974 Hanes Survey

Height	Age Group in Years 18-24	25-34	35-44	45-54	54-64	65-74
			(Weight in Pounds)			
Females:						
57"	114	118	125	129	132	130
58"	117	121	129	133	136	134
59"	120	125	133	136	140	137
60"	123	128	137	140	143	140
61"	126	132	141	143	147	144
62"	129	136	144	147	150	147
63"	132	139	148	150	153	151
64"	135	142	152	154	157	154
65"	138	146	156	158	160	158
66"	141	150	159	161	164	161
67"	144	153	163	165	167	165
68"	147	157	167	168	171	169
Males:						
62"	130	141	143	147	143	143
63"	135	145	148	152	147	147
64"	140	150	153	156	153	151
65"	145	156	158	160	158	156
66"	150	160	163	164	163	160
67"	154	165	169	169	168	164
68"	159	170	174	173	173	169
69"	164	174	179	177	178	173
70"	168	179	184	182	183	177
71"	173	184	190	187	189	182
72"	178	189	194	191	193	186
73"	183	194	200	196	197	190
74"	188	199	205	200	203	194

Note: Examined persons were measured without shoes; clothing weight ranged from 0.20 to 0.62 lb. which was not deducted from weight shown.

Adapted from Table 4 and 5, Weight by Height and Age of Adults 18-74 Years: United States, 1971-1974, DHEW Series 11, No. 208, 1979. Center for Disease Control, Atlanta, GA.

* Expected means.

METROPOLITAN LIFE INSURANCE WEIGHT STANDARDS

To Make an Approximation of Your Frame Size...

Extend your arm and bend the forearm upward at a 90 degree angle. Keep fingers straight and turn the inside of your wrist toward your body. If you have a caliper, use it to measure the space between the two prominent bones on either side of your elbow. Without a caliper, place thumb and index finger of your other hand on these two bones. Measure the space between your fingers against a ruler or tape measure. Compare it with these tables that list elbow measurements for medium-framed men and women. Measurements lower than those listed indicate you have a small frame. Higher measurements indicate a large frame.

Height in 1" heels	Elbow Breadth
MEN	
5'2" - 5'3"	2-1/2" - 2-7/8"
5'4" - 5'7"	2-5/8" - 2-7/8"
5'8" - 5'11"	2-3/4" - 3"
6'0" - 6'3"	2-3/4" - 3-1/8"
6'4"	2-7/8" - 3-1/4"
WOMEN	
4'10" - 4'11"	2-1/4" - 2-1/2"
5'0" - 5'3"	2-1/4" - 2-1/2"
5'4" - 5'7"	2-3/8" - 2-5/8"
5'8" - 5'11"	2-3/8" - 2-5/8"
6'0"	2-1/2" - 2-3/4"

1983 Metropolitan Height and Weight Tables

MEN

Height Feet	Height Inches	Small Frame	Medium Frame	Large Frame
5	2	128-134	131-141	138-150
5	3	130-136	133-143	140-153
5	4	132-138	135-145	142-156
5	5	134-140	137-148	144-160
5	6	136-142	139-151	146-164
5	7	138-145	142-154	149-168
5	8	140-148	145-157	152-172
5	9	142-151	148-160	155-176
5	10	144-154	151-163	158-180
5	11	146-157	154-166	161-184
6	0	149-160	157-170	164-188
6	1	152-164	160-174	168-192
6	2	155-168	164-178	172-197
6	3	158-172	167-182	176-202
6	4	162-176	171-187	181-207

WOMEN

Height Feet	Height Inches	Small Frame	Medium Frame	Large Frame
4	10	102-111	109-121	118-131
4	11	103-113	111-123	120-134
5	0	104-115	113-126	122-137
5	1	106-118	115-129	125-140
5	2	108-121	118-132	128-143
5	3	111-124	121-135	131-147
5	4	114-127	124-138	134-151
5	5	117-130	127-141	137-155
5	6	120-133	130-144	140-159
5	7	123-136	133-147	143-163
5	8	126-139	136-150	146-167
5	9	129-142	139-153	149-170
5	10	132-145	142-156	152-173
5	11	135-148	145-159	155-176
6	0	138-151	148-162	158-179

U.S. Recommended Daily Allowances (U.S. RDAs)[1]

	ADULTS AND CHILDREN 4 OR MORE YEARS OF AGE (For use in labeling conventional foods and also for "special dietary foods.")	INFANTS AND CHILDREN UNDER 4 YEARS OF AGE (For use only with "special dietary foods.")	PREGNANT OR LACTATING WOMEN
Nutrients Which Must Be Declared on the Label (in the order below)			
Protein[2]	45 gm "high quality protein" 65 gm "protein in general"	________	________
Vitamin A	5,000 I.U.	2,500 I.U.	8,000 I.U.
Vitamin C (or ascorbic acid)	60 mg	40 mg	60 mg
Thiamin (or Vitamin B_1)	1.5 mg	0.7 mg	1.7 mg
Riboflavin (or Vitamin B_2)	1.7 mg	0.8 mg	2.0 mg
Niacin	20 mg	9 mg	20 mg
Calcium	1.0 mg	0.8 mg	1.3 mg
Iron	18 mg	10 mg	18 mg
Nutrients Which May Be Declared on the Label (in the order below)			
Vitamin D	400 I.U.	400 I.U.	400 I.U.
Vitamin E	30 I.U.	10 I.U.	30 I.U.
Vitamin B_6	2.0 mg	0.7 mg	2.5 mg
Folic Acid (or folacin)	0.4 mg	0.2 mg	0.8 mg
Vitamin B_{12}	6 ug	3 ug	8 ug
Phosphorus	1.0 gm	0.8 mg	1.3 gm
Iodine	150 ug	70 ug	150 ug
Magnesium	400 mg	200 mg	450 mg
Zinc[3]	15 mg	8 mg	15 mg
Copper[3]	2 mg	1 mg	2 mg
Biotin[3]	0.3 mg	0.15 mg	0.3 mg
Pantothenic acid[3]	10 mg	5 mg	10 mg

[1]The "U.S. RDA" is a new term replacing the term "minimum daily requirement" (MDR). The U.S. RDA values chosen are derived from the highest value for each nutrient given in the NAS-NRC tables except for calcium and phosphorus.

[2]"High quality protein" is defined as having a protein efficiency ratio (PER) equal to or greater than that of casein; "proteins in general" are those with a PER less than that of casein. Total protein with a PER less than 20% that of easein are considered "not a significant source of protein" and would not be expressed on the label in terms of the U.S. RDA but only as amount per serving.

[3]There are no NAS-NRC RDAs for biotin, pantothenic acid, zinc and copper.

Cited References

Feeney, R., P. Criner, and B. Watt: Cholesterol content of foods. Journal of the American Dietetic Association, 61: 135-148, 1972.

Frisancho, A.R.: Triceps skin fold and upper arm muscle size norms for assessment of nutritional status. American Journal of Clinical Nutrition, 27, 1052-58, 1974.

Harris, R. and E. Karmas (editors): Nutritional Evaluation of Food Processing, 2nd edition, AVI Publishing Company, 1975.

Krehl, W. and R. Winters: Effects of cooking methods on retention of vitamins and minerals in vegetables. Journal of the American Dietetic Association, 26: 966, 1950.

National Research Council: Recommended Dietary Allowances, 9th edition, Washington: NAS-NAC, 1980.

Pennington, and H. Church: Food Values of Portions Commonly Used, Philadelphia: J.B. Lippencott Company, 1980.

Ross Labs: Nutritional analysis of fast foods. Ross Timesaver Dietetic Currents, Columbus: Ross Labs, 1980.

U.S.D.A.: Composition of Foods, Handbook No. 8-1 through 8-9, Washington: U.S. Printing Office, 1973.

U.S.D.A.: Food Composition Data-Food Names and Identification Numbers--for Nutritive Value of American Foods in Common Units, Handbook No. 456, Maryland: Maryland Research Service, 1977.

U.S.D.A.: Nutritive Value of American Foods in Common Units, Handbook No. 456, Washington: U.S. Printing Office, 1975.

U.S.D.A.: Nutritive Value of Foods, Home and Garden Bulletin No. 72, Washington: U.S. Printing Office, 1975.

TABLE 1. NUTRITIONAL ANALYSES OF FAST FOODS

(Dashes indicate no data available. X = Less than 2% US RDA; tr = trace.)

							Vitamins								Minerals									
	Wt (g)	Energy (kcal)	PRO (g)	CHO (g)	Fat (g)	Chol (mg)	A (IU)	B_1 (mg)	B_2 (mg)	Nia. (mg)	B_6 (mg)	B_{12} (μg)	C (mg)	D (IU)	Ca (mg)	Cu (mg)	Fe (mg)	K (mg)	Mg (mg)	P (mg)	Na (mg)	Zn (mg)	Moisture (g)	Crude Fiber (g)
ARBY'S®																								
Roast Beef	140	350	22	32	15	45	X	0.30	0.34	5	-	-	X	-	80	-	3.6	-	-	-	880	-	-	-
Beef and Cheese	168	450	27	36	22	55	X	0.38	0.43	6	-	-	X	-	200	-	4.5	-	-	-	1220	-	-	-
Super Roast Beef	263	620	30	61	28	85	X	0.53	0.43	7	-	-	X	-	100	-	5.4	-	-	-	1420	-	-	-
Junior Roast Beef	74	220	12	21	9	35	X	0.15	0.17	3	-	-	X	-	40	-	1.8	-	-	-	530	-	-	-
Ham & Cheese	154	380	23	33	17	60	X	0.75	0.34	5	-	-	X	-	200	-	2.7	-	-	-	1350	-	-	-
Turkey Deluxe	236	510	28	46	24	70	X	0.45	0.34	8	-	-	X	-	80	-	2.7	-	-	-	1220	-	-	-
Club Sandwich	252	560	30	43	30	100	X	0.68	0.43	7	-	-	X	-	200	-	3.6	-	-	-	1610	-	-	-

Source: Consumer Affairs, Arby's Inc., Atlanta, Georgia. Nutritional analysis by Technological Resources, Camden, New Jersey.

	Wt (g)	Energy (kcal)	PRO (g)	CHO (g)	Fat (g)	Chol (mg)	A (IU)	B_1 (mg)	B_2 (mg)	Nia. (mg)	B_6 (mg)	B_{12} (μg)	C (mg)	D (IU)	Ca (mg)	Cu (mg)	Fe (mg)	K (mg)	Mg (mg)	P (mg)	Na (mg)	Zn (mg)	Moisture (g)	Crude Fiber (g)
BURGER CHEF®																								
Hamburger	91	244	11	29	9	27	114	0.17	0.16	2.7	0.16	0.26	1.2	-	45	0.08	2.0	208	9	106	-	1.6	41	0.2
Cheeseburger	104	290	14	29	13	39	267	0.18	0.21	2.8	0.17	0.36	1.2	-	132	0.08	2.2	218	9	202	-	1.9	46	0.2
Double Cheeseburger	145	420	24	30	22	77	431	0.20	0.32	4.4	0.31	0.73	1.2	-	223	0.10	3.2	360	15	355	-	3.6	67	0.2
Fish Filet	179	547	21	46	31	43	400	0.23	0.22	2.7	0.04	0.10	1.0	-	145	0.04	2.2	271	19	302	-	1.2	72	0.4
Super Shef® Sandwich	252	563	29	44	30	105	754	0.31	0.40	6.0	0.45	0.87	9.3	-	205	0.21	4.5	578	25	377	-	4.5	143	0.5
Big Shef® Sandwich	186	569	23	38	36	81	279	0.26	0.31	4.7	0.31	0.63	1.0	-	152	0.05	3.6	382	14	280	-	3.4	80	0.3
TOP Shef® Sandwich	138	661	41	36	38	134	273	0.35	0.47	8.1	0.56	1.16	0	-	194	0.13	5.4	612	26	445	-	5.9	91	0.1
Funmeal® Feast	-	545	15	55	30	27	123	0.25	0.21	4.6	0.16	0.26	12.8	-	61	0.24	2.8	688	26	183	-	1.6	70	0.8
Rancher® Platter*	316	640	32	33	42	106	1750*	0.29	0.38	8.6	0.61	1.01	23.5	-	66	0.38	5.3	1237	53	326	-	5.6	209	1.3
Mariner™ Platter*	373	734	29	78	34	35	2069*	0.34	0.23	5.2	0.09	0.56	23.5	-	63	0.32	3.3	996	49	397	-	1.2	195	1.8
French Fries, small	68	250	2	20	19	0	0	0.07	0.04	1.7	-	0	11.5	-	9	0.16	0.7	473	16	62	-	<0.1	29	0.6
French Fries, large	85	351	3	28	26	0	0	0.10	0.06	2.4	-	0	16.2	-	13	0.23	0.9	661	22	86	-	<0.1	40	0.9
Vanilla Shake (12 oz)	336	380	13	60	10	40	387	0.10	0.66	0.5	0.1	1.77	0	-	497	-	0.3	622	40	392	-	1.3	-	-
Chocolate Shake (12 oz)	336	403	10	72	9	36	292	0.16	0.76	0.4	0.1	1.07	0	-	449	-	1.1	762	54	429	-	1.6	-	-
Hot Chocolate	-	198	8	23	8	30	288	0.93	0.39	0.3	0.1	0.79	2.1	-	271	0.09	0.7	436	50	245	-	1.1	-	-

*Includes salad. Source: Burger Chef Systems, Inc., Indianapolis, Indiana. Nutritional analysis from Handbook No. 8. Washington: US Dept. of Agriculture.

	Wt (g)	Energy (kcal)	PRO (g)	CHO (g)	Fat (g)	Chol (mg)	A (IU)	B_1 (mg)	B_2 (mg)	Nia. (mg)	B_6 (mg)	B_{12} (μg)	C (mg)	D (IU)	Ca (mg)	Cu (mg)	Fe (mg)	K (mg)	Mg (mg)	P (mg)	Na (mg)	Zn (mg)	Moisture (g)	Crude Fiber (g)
CHURCH'S FRIED CHICKEN®																								
White Chicken Portion	100	327	21	10	23	-	160	0.10	0.18	7.2	-	-	0.7	-	94	-	1.00	186	-	-	498	-	45	0.1
Dark Chicken Portion	100	305	22	7	21	-	140	0.10	0.27	5.3	-	-	1.0	-	15	-	1.3	206	-	-	475	-	48	0.2

Source: Church's Fried Chicken, San Antonio, Texas. Nutritional analysis by Medallion Laboratories, Minneapolis, Minnesota.

	Wt (g)	Energy (kcal)	PRO (g)	CHO (g)	Fat (g)	Chol (mg)	A (IU)	B_1 (mg)	B_2 (mg)	Nia. (mg)	B_6 (mg)	B_{12} (μg)	C (mg)	D (IU)	Ca (mg)	Cu (mg)	Fe (mg)	K (mg)	Mg (mg)	P (mg)	Na (mg)	Zn (mg)	Moisture (g)	Crude Fiber (g)
DAIRY QUEEN®																								
Frozen Dessert	113	180	5	27	6	20	100	0.09	0.17	X	-	0.6	X	-	150	-	X	-	-	100	-	-	-	-
DQ Cone, small	71	110	3	18	3	10	100	0.03	0.14	X	-	0.4	X	X	100	-	X	-	-	60	-	-	-	-
DQ Cone, regular	142	230	6	35	7	20	300	0.09	0.26	X	-	0.6	X	X	200	-	X	-	-	150	-	-	-	-
DQ Cone, large	213	340	10	52	10	30	400	0.15	0.43	X	-	1.2	X	8	300	-	X	-	-	200	-	-	-	-
DQ Dip Cone, small	78	150	3	20	7	10	100	0.03	0.17	X	-	0.4	X	X	100	-	X	-	-	80	-	-	-	-
DQ Dip Cone, regular	156	300	7	40	13	20	300	0.09	0.34	X	-	0.6	X	X	200	-	0.4	-	-	150	-	-	-	-
DQ Dip Cone, large	234	450	10	58	20	30	400	0.12	0.51	X	-	0.9	X	8	300	-	0.4	-	-	200	-	-	-	-
DQ Sundae, small	106	170	4	30	4	15	100	0.03	0.17	X	-	0.5	X	X	100	-	0.7	-	-	100	-	-	-	-
DQ Sundae, regular	177	290	6	51	7	20	300	0.06	0.26	X	-	0.6	X	X	200	-	1.1	-	-	150	-	-	-	-
DQ Sundae, large	248	400	9	71	9	30	400	0.09	0.43	0.4	-	1.2	X	8	300	-	1.8	-	-	250	-	-	-	-
DQ Malt, small	241	340	10	51	11	30	400	0.06	0.34	0.4	-	1.2	2.4	60	300	-	1.8	-	-	200	-	-	-	-
DQ Malt, regular	418	600	15	89	20	50	750	0.12	0.60	0.8	-	1.8	3.6	100	500	-	3.6	-	-	400	-	-	-	-
DQ Malt, large	588	840	22	125	28	70	750	0.15	0.85	1.2	-	2.4	6	140	600	-	5.4	-	-	600	-	-	-	-
DQ Float	397	330	6	59	8	20	100	0.12	0.17	X	-	0.6	X	X	200	-	X	-	-	200	-	-	-	-
DQ Banana Split	383	540	10	91	15	30	750	0.60	0.60	0.8	-	0.9	18	X	350	-	1.8	-	-	250	-	-	-	-
DQ Parfait	284	460	10	81	11	30	400	0.12	0.43	0.4	-	1.2	X	8	300	-	1.8	-	-	250	-	-	-	-
DQ Freeze	397	520	11	89	13	35	200	0.15	0.34	X	-	1.2	X	X	300	-	X	-	-	250	-	-	-	-
Mr. Misty® Freeze	411	500	10	87	12	35	200	0.15	0.34	X	-	0.12	X	X	300	-	X	-	-	200	-	-	-	-
Mr. Misty® Float	404	440	6	85	8	20	100	0.12	0.17	X	-	0.6	X	X	200	-	X	-	-	200	-	-	-	-

TABLE 1. NUTRITIONAL ANALYSES OF FAST FOODS

(Dashes indicate no data available. X = Less than 2% US RDA; tr = trace.)

	Wt (g)	Energy (kcal)	PRO (g)	CHO (g)	Fat (g)	Chol (mg)	Vitamins A (IU)	B_1 (mg)	B_2 (mg)	Nia. (mg)	B_6 (mg)	B_{12} (μg)	C (mg)	D (IU)	Minerals Ca (mg)	Cu (mg)	Fe (mg)	K (mg)	Mg (mg)	P (mg)	Na (mg)	Zn (mg)	Moisture (g)	Crude Fiber (g)
"Dilly"® Bar	85	240	4	22	15	10	100	0.06	0.17	X	-	0.5	X	X	100	-	0.4	-	-	100	-	-	-	-
DQ Sandwich	60	140	3	24	4	10	100	0.03	0.14	0.4	-	0.2	X	X	60	-	0.4	-	-	60	-	-	-	-
Mr. Misty Kiss®	89	70	0	17	0	0	X	X	X	X	-	X	X	X	X	-	X	-	-	X	-	-	-	-
Brazier® Cheese Dog	113	330	15	24	19	-	-	-	0.18	3.3	0.07	1.22	-	23	168	0.08	1.6	-	24	182	-	1.9	-	-
Brazier® Chili Dog	128	330	13	25	20	-	-	0.15	0.23	3.9	0.17	1.29	11.0	20	86	0.13	2.0	-	38	139	939	1.8	-	-
Brazier® Dog	99	273	11	23	15	-	-	0.12	0.15	2.6	0.08	1.05	11.0	23	75	0.79	1.5	-	21	104	868	1.4	-	-
Fish Sandwich	170	400	20	41	17	-	tr	0.15	0.26	3.0	0.16	1.20	tr	40	60	0.08	1.1	-	24	200	-	0.3	-	-
Fish Sandwich w/Ch	177	440	24	39	21	-	100	0.15	0.26	3.0	0.16	1.50	tr	40	150	0.08	0.4	-	24	250	-	0.3	-	-
Super Brazier® Dog	182	518	20	41	30	-	tr	0.42	0.44	7.0	0.17	2.09	14.0	44	158	0.18	4.3	-	37	195	1552	2.8	-	-
Super Brazier® Dog w/Ch	203	593	26	43	36	-	-	0.43	0.48	8.1	0.18	2.34	14.0	44	297	0.18	4.4	-	42	312	1986	3.5	-	-
Super Brazier® Chili Dog	210	555	23	42	33	-	-	0.42	0.48	8.8	0.27	2.67	18.0	32	158	0.21	4.0	-	48	231	1640	2.8	-	-
Brazier® Fries, small	71	200	2	25	10	-	tr	0.06	tr	0.8	0.16	-	3.6	16	tr	0.04	0.4	-	16	100	-	tr	-	-
Brazier® Fried, large	113	320	3	40	16	-	tr	0.09	0.03	1.2	0.30	-	4.8	24	tr	0.08	0.4	-	24	150	-	0.3	-	-
Brazier® Onion Rings	85	300	6	33	17	-	tr	0.09	tr	0.4	0.08	-	2.4	8	20	0.08	0.4	-	16	60	-	0.3	-	-

Source: International Dairy Queen, Inc., Minneapolis, Minnesota. Nutritional analysis by Raltech Scientific Services, Inc. (formerly WARF), Madison, Wisconsin. (Nutritional analysis not applicable in the state of Texas.)

	Wt (g)	Energy (kcal)	PRO (g)	CHO (g)	Fat (g)	Chol (mg)	A (IU)	B_1 (mg)	B_2 (mg)	Nia. (mg)	B_6 (mg)	B_{12} (μg)	C (mg)	D (IU)	Ca (mg)	Cu (mg)	Fe (mg)	K (mg)	Mg (mg)	P (mg)	Na (mg)	Zn (mg)	Moisture (g)	Crude Fiber (g)
JACK IN THE BOX®																								
Hamburger	97	263	13	29	11	26	49	0.27	0.18	5.6	0.11	0.73	1.1	20	82	0.10	2.3	165	20	115	566	1.8	43	0.2
Cheeseburger	109	310	16	28	15	32	338	0.27	0.21	5.5	0.12	0.87	<1.1	20	172	0.10	2.6	177	22	194	877	2.3	47	0.2
Jumbo Jack® Hamburger	246	551	28	45	29	80	246	0.47	0.34	11.6	0.30	2.68	3.7	42	134	0.22	4.5	492	44	261	1134	4.2	139	0.7
Jumbo Jack® Hamburger w/Ch	272	628	32	45	35	110	734	0.52	0.38	11.3	0.31	3.05	4.9	41	273	0.24	4.6	499	49	411	1666	4.8	153	0.8
Regular Taco	83	189	8	15	11	22	356	0.07	0.08	1.8	0.14	0.5	<0.9	6	116	0.11	1.2	264	36	150	460	1.3	47	0.6
Super Taco	146	285	12	20	17	37	599	0.10	0.12	2.8	0.22	0.77	1.6	9	196	0.18	1.9	415	53	235	968	2.1	92	1.0
Moby Jack® Sandwich	141	455	17	38	26	56	240	0.30	0.21	4.5	0.12	1.1	1.4	24	167	0.08	1.7	246	30	263	837	1.1	57	0.1
Breakfast Jack® Sandwich	121	301	18	28	13	182	442	0.41	0.47	5.1	0.14	1.1	3.4	51	177	0.11	2.5	190	24	310	1037	1.8	59	0.1
French Fries	80	270	3	31	15	13	-	0.12	0.02	1.9	0.22	0.17	3.7	<1	19	0.10	0.7	423	27	88	128	0.3	29	0.6
Onion Rings	85	351	5	32	23	24	-	0.24	0.12	3.1	0.07	0.26	<1.2	<1	26	0.07	1.4	109	16	69	318	0.4	24	0.3
Apple Turnover	119	411	4	45	24	17	-	0.23	0.12	2.5	0.03	0.17	<1.2	1	11	0.06	1.4	69	10	33	352	0.2	45	0.2
Vanilla Shake*	317	317	10	57	6	26	-	0.16	0.38	0.5	0.20	1.36	<3.2	41	349	0.06	0.2	599	38	312	229	1.0	243	0.3
Strawberry Shake*	328	323	11	55	7	26	-	0.16	0.46	0.6	0.15	1.25	<3.3	43	371	0.10	0.6	613	40	328	241	1.1	253	0.3
Chocolate Shake*	322	325	11	55	7	26	-	0.16	0.64	0.6	0.19	1.55	<3.2	45	348	0.13	0.7	676	53	328	270	1.1	247	0.3
Vanilla Shake	314	342	10	54	9	36	440	0.16	0.47	0.5	0.18	1.1	3.5	44	349	0.06	0.4	536	48	318	263	1.0	238	0.3
Strawberry Shake	328	380	11	63	10	33	426	0.16	0.62	0.5	0.18	0.92	<3.3	30	351	0.07	0.3	556	47	316	268	1.0	242	0.3
Chocolate Shake	317	365	11	59	10	35	380	0.16	0.60	0.6	0.18	0.98	<3.2	38	350	0.16	1.2	633	57	332	294	1.2	235	0.3
Ham & Cheese Omelette	174	425	21	32	23	355	766	0.45	0.70	3.0	0.18	1.44	<1.7	64	260	0.14	4.0	237	29	397	975	2.3	94	0.2
Double Cheese Omelette	166	423	19	30	25	370	797	0.33	0.68	2.5	0.14	1.33	1.7	61	276	0.13	3.6	208	26	370	899	2.1	88	0.2
Ranchero Style Omelette	196	414	20	33	23	343	853	0.33	0.74	2.6	0.18	1.51	<2.0	78	278	0.14	3.8	260	29	372	1098	2.0	117	0.4
French Toast	180	537	15	54	29	115	522	0.56	0.30	4.4	0.47	1.62	9.2	22	119	0.11	3.0	194	27	256	1130	1.8	78	0.9
Pancakes	232	626	16	79	27	87	488	0.63	0.44	4.6	0.19	0.56	<26.1	23	105	0.12	2.8	237	36	633	1670	1.9	104	0.7
Scrambled Eggs	267	719	26	55	44	259	694	0.69	0.56	5.2	0.34	1.31	<12.8	80	257	0.24	5.0	635	55	483	1110	3.0	137	1.3

*Special Formula for shakes sold in California, Arizona, Texas and Washington. Source: Jack-in-the-Box, Foodmaker, Inc., San Diego, California. Nutritional analysis by Raltech Scientific Services, Inc. (formerly WARF), Madison, Wisconsin.

	Wt (g)	Energy (kcal)	PRO (g)	CHO (g)	Fat (g)	Chol (mg)	A (IU)	B_1 (mg)	B_2 (mg)	Nia. (mg)	B_6 (mg)	B_{12} (μg)	C (mg)	D (IU)	Ca (mg)	Cu (mg)	Fe (mg)	K (mg)	Mg (mg)	P (mg)	Na (mg)	Zn (mg)	Moisture (g)	Crude Fiber (g)
KENTUCKY FRIED CHICKEN®																								
Original Recipe® Dinner*																								
Wing & Rib	322	603	30	48	32	133	25.5	0.22	0.19	10.0	-	-	36.6	-	-	-	-	-	-	-	-	-	-	-
Wing & Thigh	341	661	33	48	38	172	25.5	0.24	0.27	8.4	-	-	36.6	-	-	-	-	-	-	-	-	-	-	-
Drum & Thigh	346	643	35	46	35	180	25.5	0.25	0.32	8.5	-	-	36.6	-	-	-	-	-	-	-	-	-	-	-
Extra Crispy Dinner*																								
Wing & Rib	349	755	33	60	43	132	25.5	0.31	0.29	10.4	-	-	36.6	-	-	-	-	-	-	-	-	-	-	-
Wing & Thigh	371	812	36	58	48	176	25.5	0.31	0.35	10.3	-	-	36.6	-	-	-	-	-	-	-	-	-	-	-
Drum & Thigh	376	765	38	55	44	183	25.5	0.32	0.38	10.4	-	-	36.6	-	-	-	-	-	-	-	-	-	-	-
Mashed Potatoes	85	64	2	12	1	0	<18	<0.01	0.02	0.8	-	-	4.9	-	-	-	-	-	-	-	-	-	-	-
Gravy	14	23	0	1	2	0	< 3	0.00	0.01	0.1	-	-	<0.2	-	-	-	-	-	-	-	-	-	-	-
Cole Slaw	91	122	1	13	8	7	-	-	-	-	-	-	-	-	-	-	-	-	-	-	-	-	-	-
Rolls	21	61	2	11	1	1	< 5	0.10	0.04	1.0	-	-	0.3	-	-	-	-	-	-	-	-	-	-	-
Corn (5.5 inch ear)	135	169	5	31	3	X	162	0.12	0.07	1.2	-	-	2.6	-	-	-	-	-	-	-	-	-	-	-

*Includes two pieces of chicken, mashed potato and gravy, cole slaw, and roll. Source: Kentucky Fried Chicken, Inc., Louisville, Kentucky. Nutritional analysis by Raltech Services, Inc. (formerly WARF), Madison, Wisconsin.

TABLE 1. NUTRITIONAL ANALYSES OF FAST FOODS

(Dashes indicate no data available. X = Less than 2% US RDA; tr = trace.)

	Wt (g)	Energy (kcal)	PRO (g)	CHO (g)	Fat (g)	Chol (mg)	Vitamins A (IU)	B_1 (mg)	B_2 (mg)	Nia. (mg)	B_6 (mg)	B_{12} (μg)	C (mg)	D (IU)	Minerals Ca (mg)	Cu (mg)	Fe (mg)	K (mg)	Mg (mg)	P (mg)	Na (mg)	Zn (mg)	Mois-ture (g)	Crude Fiber (g)
LONG JOHN SILVER'S®																								
Fish w/Batter (2 pc)	136	366	22	21	22	-	-	-	-	-	-	-	-	-	-	-	-	-	-	-	-	-	-	-
Fish w/Batter (3 pc)	207	549	32	32	32	-	-	-	-	-	-	-	-	-	-	-	-	-	-	-	-	-	-	-
Treasure Chest™	143	506	30	32	33	-	-	-	-	-	-	-	-	-	-	-	-	-	-	-	-	-	-	-
Chicken Planks® (4 pc)	166	457	27	35	23	-	-	-	-	-	-	-	-	-	-	-	-	-	-	-	-	-	-	-
Peg Legs™ w/Batter (5 pc)	125	350	22	26	28	-	-	-	-	-	-	-	-	-	-	-	-	-	-	-	-	-	-	-
Ocean Scallops (6 pc)	120	283	11	30	13	-	-	-	-	-	-	-	-	-	-	-	-	-	-	-	-	-	-	-
Shrimp w/Batter (6 pc)	88	268	8	30	13	-	-	-	-	-	-	-	-	-	-	-	-	-	-	-	-	-	-	-
Breaded Oysters (6 pc)	156	441	13	53	19	-	-	-	-	-	-	-	-	-	-	-	-	-	-	-	-	-	-	-
Breaded Clams	142	617	18	61	34	-	-	-	-	-	-	-	-	-	-	-	-	-	-	-	-	-	-	-
Fish Sandwich	193	337	22	49	31	-	-	-	-	-	-	-	-	-	-	-	-	-	-	-	-	-	-	-
French Fryes	85	288	4	33	16	-	-	-	-	-	-	-	-	-	-	-	-	-	-	-	-	-	-	-
Cole Slaw	113	138	1	16	8	-	-	-	-	-	-	-	-	-	-	-	-	-	-	-	-	-	-	-
Corn on the Cob (1 ear)	150	176	5	29	4	-	-	-	-	-	-	-	-	-	-	-	-	-	-	-	-	-	-	-
Hushpuppies (3)	45	153	3	20	7	-	-	-	-	-	-	-	-	-	-	-	-	-	-	-	-	-	-	-
Clam Chowder (8 oz)	170	107	5	15	3	-	-	-	-	-	-	-	-	-	-	-	-	-	-	-	-	-	-	-

Source: Long John Silver's Food Shoppes, Lexington, Kentucky. Nutritional analysis by L. V. Packett, Ph.D. The Department of Nutrition and Science, University of Kentucky.

	Wt (g)	Energy (kcal)	PRO (g)	CHO (g)	Fat (g)	Chol (mg)	A (IU)	B_1 (mg)	B_2 (mg)	Nia. (mg)	B_6 (mg)	B_{12} (μg)	C (mg)	D (IU)	Ca (mg)	Cu (mg)	Fe (mg)	K (mg)	Mg (mg)	P (mg)	Na (mg)	Zn (mg)	Mois-ture (g)	Crude Fiber (g)
McDONALD'S®																								
Egg McMuffin®	138	327	19	31	15	229	97	0.47	0.44	3.8	0.21	0.75	<1.4	46	226	0.12	2.9	168	26	322	885	1.9	70.7	0.1
English Muffin, Buttered	63	186	5	30	5	13	164	0.28	0.49	2.6	0.04	0.02	0.8	14	117	0.69	1.5	71	13	74	318	0.5	21.7	0.1
Hotcakes w/Butter & Syrup	214	500	8	94	10	47	257	0.26	0.36	2.3	0.12	0.19	4.7	5	103	0.11	2.2	187	28	501	1070	0.7	97.8	0.2
Sausage (Pork)	53	206	9	tr	19	43	<32	0.27	0.11	2.1	0.18	0.53	0.5	31	16	0.05	0.8	127	9	95	615	1.5	22.9	0.1
Scrambled Eggs	98	180	13	3	13	349	652	0.08	0.47	0.2	0.19	0.93	1.2	65	61	0.06	2.5	135	13	264	205	1.7	68.1	<0.1
Hashbrown Potatoes	55	125	2	14	7	7	<14	0.06	<0.01	0.8	0.13	0.01	4.1	<1	5	0.04	0.4	247	13	67	325	0.2	30.9	0.3
Big Mac®	204	563	26	41	33	86	530	0.39	0.37	6.5	0.27	1.8	2.2	33	157	0.18	4.0	237	38	314	1010	4.7	100.4	0.6
Cheeseburger	115	307	15	30	14	37	345	0.25	0.23	3.8	0.12	0.91	1.6	13	132	0.11	2.4	156	23	205	767	2.6	108.4	0.2
Hamburger	102	255	12	30	10	25	82	0.25	0.18	4.0	0.12	0.81	1.7	12	51	0.10	2.3	142	19	126	520	2.1	48.0	0.3
Quarter Pounder®	166	424	24	33	22	67	133	0.32	0.28	6.5	0.27	1.88	<1.7	23	63	0.17	4.1	322	37	249	735	5.1	83.7	0.7
Quarter Pounder® w/Ch	194	524	30	32	31	96	660	0.31	0.37	7.4	0.23	2.15	2.7	25	219	0.18	4.3	341	41	382	1236	5.7	96.0	0.8
Filet-O-Fish®	139	432	14	37	25	47	42	0.26	0.20	2.6	0.10	0.82	<1.4	25	93	0.10	1.7	150	27	229	781	0.9	59.5	0.1
Regular Fries	68	220	3	26	12	9	<17	0.12	0.02	2.3	0.22	<0.03	12.5	<1	9	0.03	0.6	564	27	101	109	0.3	25.4	0.5
Apple Pie	85	253	2	29	14	12	<34	0.02	0.02	0.2	0.02	<0.04	<0.8	2	14	0.05	0.6	39	6	27	398	0.2	38.3	0.3
Cherry Pie	88	260	2	32	14	13	114	0.03	0.02	0.4	0.02	<0.02	<0.8	<2	12	0.06	0.6	35	7	27	427	0.2	38.9	0.1
McDonaldland® Cookies	67	308	4	49	11	10	<27	0.23	0.23	2.9	0.03	0.03	0.9	10	12	0.07	1.5	52	11	74	358	0.3	2.2	0.1
Chocolate Shake	291	383	10	66	9	30	349	0.12	0.44	0.5	0.13	1.16	<2.9	44	320	0.19	0.8	580	49	335	300	1.4	203.0	0.3
Strawberry Shake	290	362	9	62	9	32	377	0.12	0.44	0.4	0.14	1.16	4.1	32	322	0.07	0.2	423	31	313	207	1.2	207.9	<0.3
Vanilla Shake	291	352	9	60	8	31	349	0.12	0.70	0.3	0.12	1.19	3.2	26	329	0.09	0.2	422	31	314	201	1.2	211.3	<0.3
Hot Fudge Sundae	164	310	7	46	11	18	230	0.07	0.31	1.1	0.13	0.7	2.5	16	215	0.13	0.6	410	35	236	175	1.0	97.9	0.2
Caramel Sundae	165	328	7	53	10	26	279	0.07	0.31	1.0	0.05	0.6	3.6	14	200	0.09	0.2	338	30	230	195	0.9	93.2	<0.2
Strawberry Sundae	164	289	7	46	9	20	230	0.07	0.30	1.0	0.05	0.6	2.8	16	174	0.11	0.4	290	28	80	96	0.8	101.0	0.2

Source: McDonald's Corporation, Oak Brook, Illinois. Nutritional analysis by Raltech Scientific Services, Inc. (formerly WARF), Madison, Wisconsin.

	Wt (g)	Energy (kcal)	PRO (g)	CHO (g)	Fat (g)	Chol (mg)	A (IU)	B_1 (mg)	B_2 (mg)	Nia. (mg)	B_6 (mg)	B_{12} (μg)	C (mg)	D (IU)	Ca (mg)	Cu (mg)	Fe (mg)	K (mg)	Mg (mg)	P (mg)	Na (mg)	Zn (mg)	Mois-ture (g)	Crude Fiber (g)
TACO BELL®																								
Bean Burrito	166	343	11	48	12	-	1657	0.37	0.22	2.2	-	-	15.2	-	98	-	2.8	235	-	173	272	-	-	-
Beef Burrito	184	466	30	37	21	-	1675	0.30	0.39	7.0	-	-	15.2	-	83	-	4.6	320	-	288	327	-	-	-
Beefy Tostada	184	291	19	21	15	-	3450	0.16	0.27	3.3	-	-	12.7	-	208	-	3.4	277	-	265	138	-	-	-
Bellbeefer®	123	221	15	23	7	-	2961	0.15	0.20	3.7	-	-	10.0	-	40	-	2.6	183	-	140	231	-	-	-
Bellbeefer® w/Ch	137	278	19	23	12	-	3146	0.16	0.27	3.7	-	-	10.0	-	147	-	2.7	195	-	208	330	-	-	-
Burrito Supreme®	225	457	21	43	22	-	3462	0.33	0.35	4.7	-	-	16.0	-	121	-	3.8	350	-	245	367	-	-	-
Combination Burrito	175	404	21	43	16	-	1666	0.34	0.31	4.6	-	-	15.2	-	91	-	3.7	278	-	230	300	-	-	-
Enchirito®	207	454	25	42	21	-	1178	0.31	0.37	4.7	-	-	9.5	-	259	-	3.8	491	-	338	1175	-	-	-
Pintos 'N Cheese	158	168	11	21	5	-	3123	0.26	0.16	0.9	-	-	9.3	-	150	-	2.3	307	-	210	102	-	-	-
Taco	83	186	15	14	8	-	120	0.09	0.16	2.9	-	-	0.2	-	120	-	2.5	143	-	175	79	-	-	-
Tostada	138	179	9	25	6	-	3152	0.18	0.15	0.8	-	-	9.7	-	191	-	2.3	172	-	186	101	-	-	-

Sources: 1) Menu Item Portions, San Antonio, Texas, Taco Bell Co., July, 1976; 2) Adams, C.F.: Nutritive value of American foods in common units in Handbook No. 456. Washington: USDA Agricultural Research Service, November 1975; 3) Church, P.F., Church, H.N. (eds) Food Values of Portions Commonly Used, ed 12, Philadelphia: J.B. Lippincott Co., 1976; 4) Valley Baptist Medical Center, Food Service Department: Fort Atkinson, Wisconsin, NASCO.

TABLE 1. NUTRITIONAL ANALYSES OF FAST FOODS

(Dashes indicate no data available. X = Less than 2% US RDA; tr = trace.)

	Wt (g)	Energy (kcal)	PRO (g)	CHO (g)	Fat (g)	Chol (mg)	Vitamins A (IU)	B_1 (mg)	B_2 (mg)	Nia. (mg)	B_6 (mg)	B_{12} (μg)	C (mg)	D (IU)	Minerals Ca (mg)	Cu (mg)	Fe (mg)	K (mg)	Mg (mg)	P (mg)	Na (mg)	Zn (mg)	Moisture (g)	Crude Fiber (g)
WENDY'S®																								
Single Hamburger	200	470	26	34	26	70	94	0.24	0.36	5.8	-	-	0.6	-	84	-	5.3	-	-	239	774	4.8	110.6	0.8
Double Hamburger	285	670	44	34	40	125	128	0.43	0.54	10.6	-	-	1.5	-	138	-	8.2	-	-	364	980	8.4	162.1	1.1
Triple Hamburger	360	850	65	33	51	205	220	0.47	0.68	14.7	-	-	2.0	-	104	-	10.7	-	-	525	1217	13.5	204.6	1.4
Single w/Cheese	240	580	33	34	34	90	221	0.38	0.43	6.3	-	-	0.7	-	228	-	5.4	-	-	315	1085	5.5	133.4	1.0
Double w/Cheese	325	800	50	41	48	155	439	0.49	0.75	11.4	-	-	2.3	-	177	-	10.2	-	-	489	1414	10.1	179.2	1.3
Triple w/Cheese	400	1040	72	35	68	225	472	0.80	0.84	15.1	-	-	3.4	-	371	-	10.9	-	-	712	1848	14.3	216.4	1.6
Chili	250	230	19	21	8	25	1188	0.22	0.25	3.4	-	-	2.9	-	83	-	4.4	-	-	168	1065	3.7	195.9	2.3
French Fries	120	330	5	41	16	5	40	0.14	0.07	3.0	-	-	6.4	-	16	-	1.2	-	-	196	112	0.5	54.9	1.2
Frosty	250	390	9	54	16	45	355	0.20	0.60	X	0	X	0.7	-	270	-	0.9	-	-	278	247	1.0	169.8	0.0

Source: Wendy's International, Inc., Dublin, Ohio. Nutritional analysis by Medallion Laboratories, Minneapolis, Minnesota.

PIZZA HUT®*

PIZZA HUT data is invalid because of reformulation of the products.

	Wt (g)	Energy (kcal)	PRO (g)	CHO (g)	Fat (g)	Chol (mg)	Vitamins A (IU)	B_1 (mg)	B_2 (mg)	Nia. (mg)	B_6 (mg)	B_{12} (μg)	C (mg)	D (IU)	Minerals Ca (mg)	Cu (mg)	Fe (mg)	K (mg)	Mg (mg)	P (mg)	Na (mg)	Zn (mg)	Moisture (g)	Crude Fiber (g)
BEVERAGES																								
Coffee*	180	2	tr	tr	tr	-	0	0	tr	0.5	-	-	0	-	4	-	0.2	65	-	7	2	-	100†	0
Tea*	180	2	tr	-	tr	-	0	0	0.04	0.1	-	-	1	-	5	-	0.2	-	-	4	-	-	40†	0
Orange Juice	183	82	1	20	tr	-	366	0.17	0.02	0.6	-	-	82.4	-	17	-	0.2	340	18	29	2	-	0	0
Chocolate Milk	250	213	9	28	9	-	330	0.08	0.40	0.3	-	-	3.0	-	278	-	0.5	365	-	235	118	-	-	0
Skim Milk	245	88	9	13	tr	-	10	0.09	0.44	0.2	-	-	2.0	-	296	-	0.1	355	-	233	127	-	-	0
Whole Milk	244	159	9	12	9	27	342	0.07	0.41	0.2	-	-	2.4	100	188	-	tr	351	32	227	122	-	-	0
Coca-Cola®	246	96	0	24	0	-	-	-	-	-	-	-	-	-	-	-	-	-	-	40	20§	-	28	0
Fanta® Ginger Ale	244	84	0	21	0	-	-	-	-	-	-	-	-	-	-	-	-	-	-	0	30§	-	0	0
Fanta® Grape	247	114	0	29	0	-	-	-	-	-	-	-	-	-	-	-	-	-	-	0	21§	-	0	0
Fanta® Orange	248	117	0	30	0	-	-	-	-	-	-	-	-	-	-	-	-	-	-	0	21§	-	0	0
Fanta® Rootbeer	246	103	0	27	0	-	-	-	-	-	-	-	-	-	-	-	-	-	-	0	23§	-	0	0
Mr. Pibb®	245	95	0	25	0	-	-	-	-	-	-	-	-	-	-	-	-	-	-	29	23§	-	27	0
Mr. Pibb® w/o Sugar	236	1	0	tr	0	-	-	-	-	-	-	-	-	-	-	-	-	-	-	28	37§	-	38	76
Sprite®	245	95	0	24	0	-	-	-	-	-	-	-	-	-	-	-	-	-	-	0	42§	-	0	0
Sprite® w/o Sugar	236	3	0	0	0	-	-	-	-	-	-	-	-	-	-	-	-	-	-	0	42§	-	0	57
Tab®	236	tr	0	tr	0	-	-	-	-	-	-	-	-	-	-	-	-	-	-	30	30§	-	30	74
Fresca®	236	2	0	0	0	-	-	-	-	-	-	-	-	-	-	-	-	-	-	0	38	-	0	54

*6-oz serving; all other data are for 8-oz serving. †Caffeine content depends on strength of beverage. §Value when bottling water with average sodium content (12 mg/8 oz) is used. Sources: 1) Adams, C.F.: Nutritive value of American foods in common units, in Handbook No. 456. Washington: USDA Agricultural Research Service, November 1975; 2) The Coca-Cola Company, Atlanta, Georgia, January 1977; 3) American Hospital Formulary Service, Washington, American Society of Hospital Pharmacists, Section 28:20, March 1978.

*[From Young, EA, UPDATE: Nutritional Analysis of Fast Foods, Dietetic Currents, 1981 (Ross Laboratories, Columbus, Ohio)]